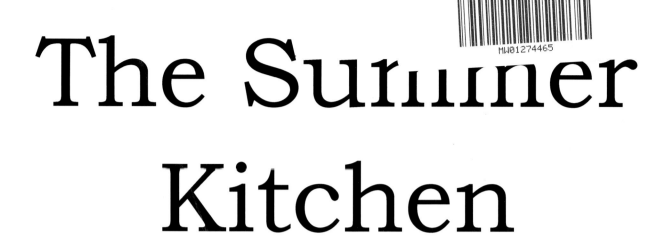

The Summer Kitchen

Rachel Vdolek

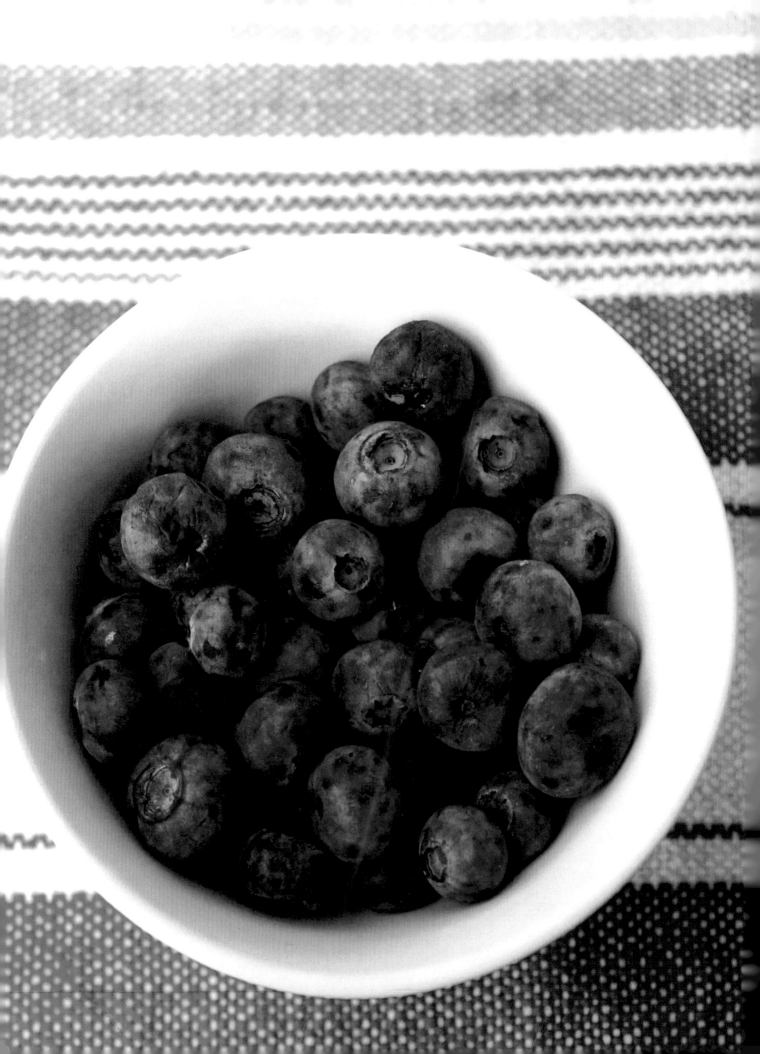

Table of Contents

Introduction 5

Summer Vegetables 6
Cucumbers 9
Green Beans 21
Lettuce 36
Summer Squash 49
Tomatoes 61
Zucchini 72

Summer Fruits 87
Apricots 88
Dark Berries 101
Cherries 112
Limes 124
Melons 137
Peaches and Nectarines 148

Allergy Notes 162
Index by dish 163
Index by secondary ingredients 165
About the author 166

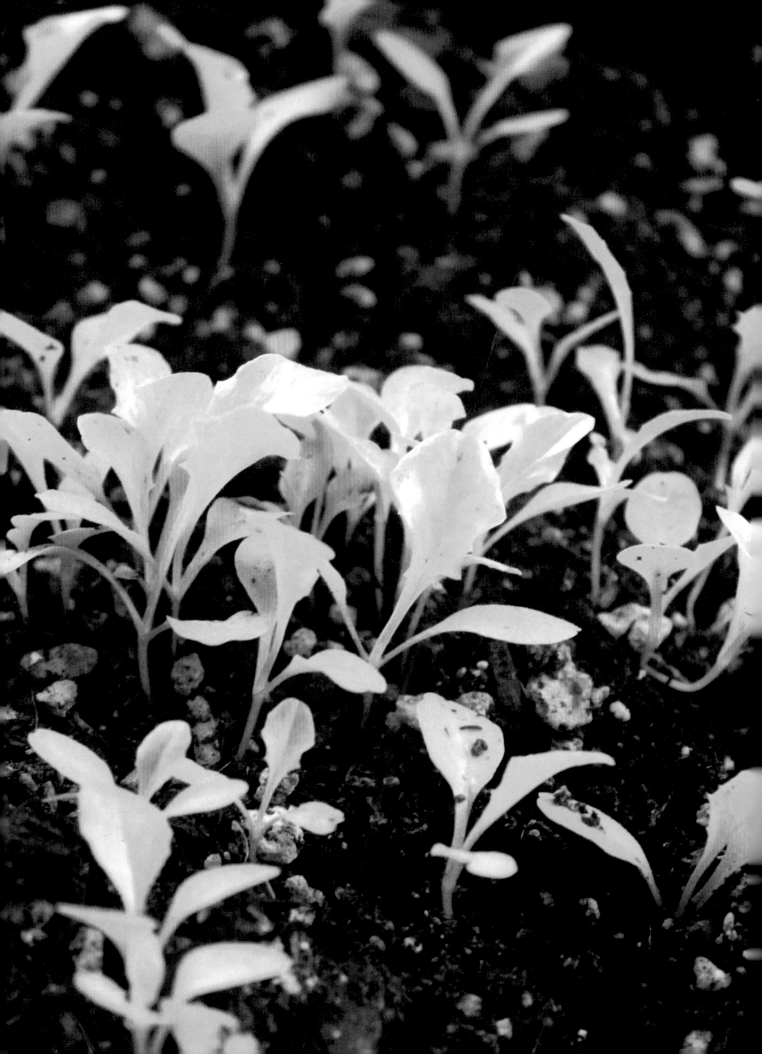

Introduction

Summer is a time of easy living, sitting in the sun, soaking up the rays. It's also a time when it gets too hot to cook and all you want is to chop, toss and eat. Summer is all about the easy, simple cooking, but it never lacks in flavor.

The recipes in this book are all based on delicious flavors that can be easily manipulated to make a wonderful dish. The produce that I have highlighted in this book include cucumbers, lettuce, green beans, zucchini, summer squash and tomatoes. All the veggie recipes are simple to make and most are great when made ahead earlier in the day when it's cooler out.

The fruits are all about keeping cool. I decided to focus this book on my favorite summer fruits, which are dark berries, nectarines and peaches, apricots, limes, cherries and melons. I combined a few together (like the blueberries and blackberries for the dark berry section) simply because I couldn't stand to not have a recipe for both in this book. The melon section especially highlights this because I have recipes for the three most popular melons: watermelon, honeydew and cantaloupe.

I hope you enjoy the recipes I have created for summer eating.

Rachel

Summer Vegetables

I love the ease of summer vegetables. Most of them don't require any cooking to get maximum flavor and those that do are ready in minutes. My favorites are tomatoes, zucchini, summer squash, cucumbers, lettuce and green beans, all of which I've included in this book.

From being grilled to baked to pickled to left in their original state, these summer vegetables are sure to be the stars of your meals during this wonderful, bountiful season.

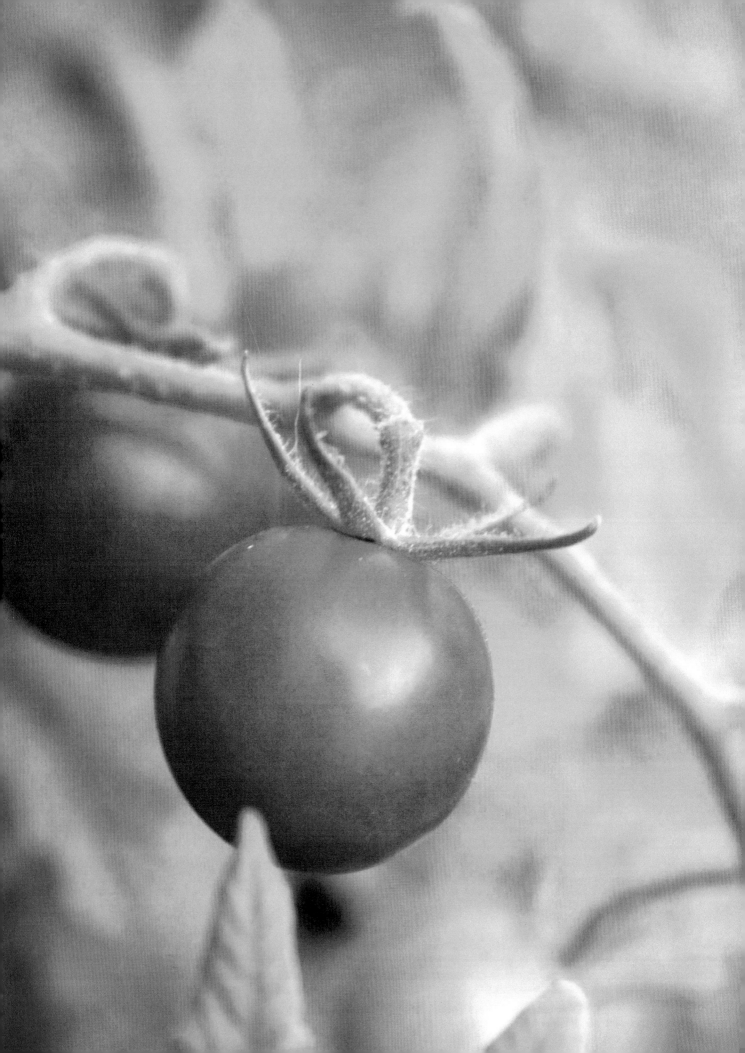

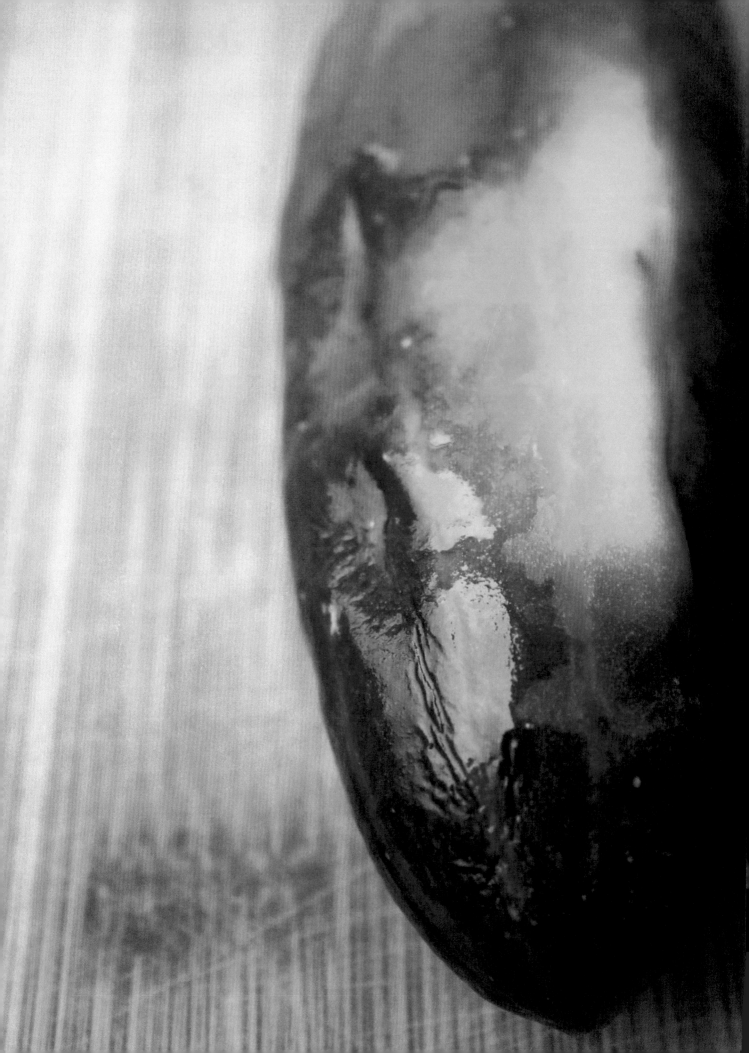

Cucumbers

The only time I ever ate cucumbers growing up was when they were pickled or put in a salad. Don't get me wrong, I love pickles (so much I even included my favorite pickle recipe in this book), but I wanted to show that cucumbers should not just be considered a condiment. They make a great cracker for any salad to be served as an appetizer, while giving any noodle salad some extra crunch.

My favorite recipe from this section is the Asian crab salad on cucumbers. They are the perfect appetizer since they are a one-bite deal. The crunch from the cucumber really pairs well with the creaminess of the crab salad. The noodles also give a little extra crunch, but the cucumber really wins it over. I ate so many of these, I couldn't even begin to tell you how many.

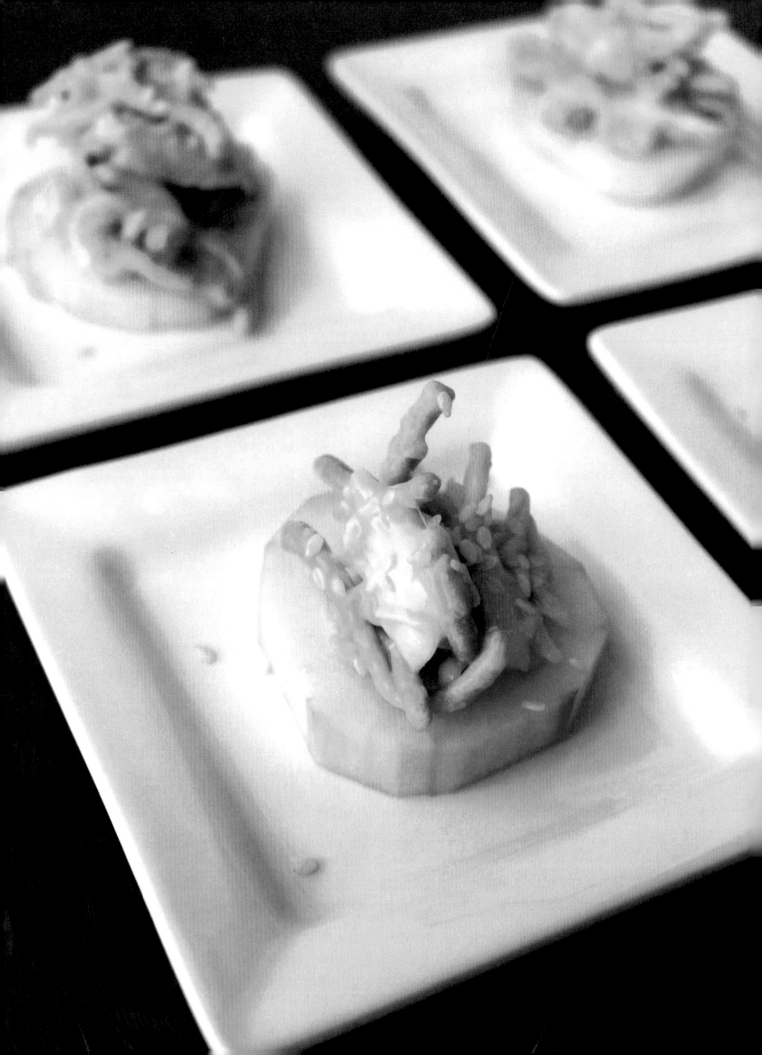

Asian Crab Salad on Cucumber Slices

Makes 12 appetizers

1/4 lb crab meat

3 tbsp mayo or vegan mayo

1 tbsp sesame oil

1 tbsp soy sauce

1/2 tsp sesame seeds

1/4 c. chow mein noodles

1 cucumber, peeled and sliced 1/2" thick

Sesame seeds, for garnish

In a medium bowl, combine all ingredients except cucumber slices. Stir to mix. Lay cucumber slices on a tray, then top each with a spoonful of the crab mixture. Sprinkle sesame seeds over the top for garnish. Serve immediately or the chow mein noodles will become soft.

Cucumber and Mint Soup

Serves 4

1 cucumber, peeled and roughly chopped

1 sprig mint

1 handful parsley

2 c. chicken or vegetable stock

1 tsp salt

½ tsp pepper

In a blender, combine all ingredients. Puree until almost smooth, then pour into a container. Cover with wrap, then chill for at least an hour to let flavors develop.

To serve, pour into small bowls or glasses.

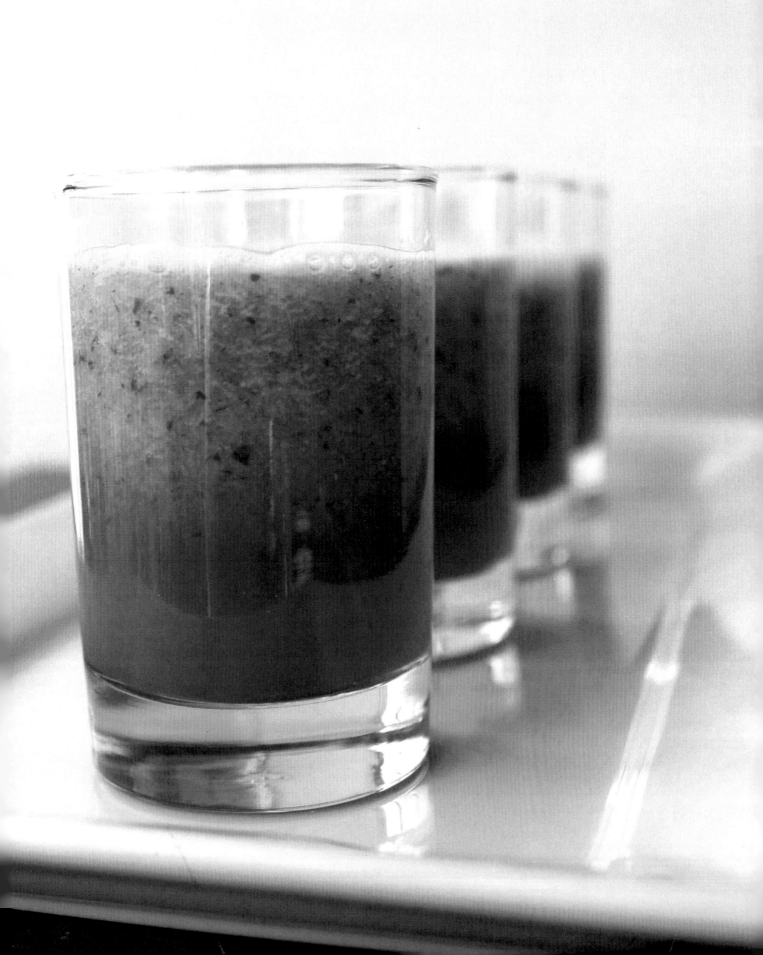

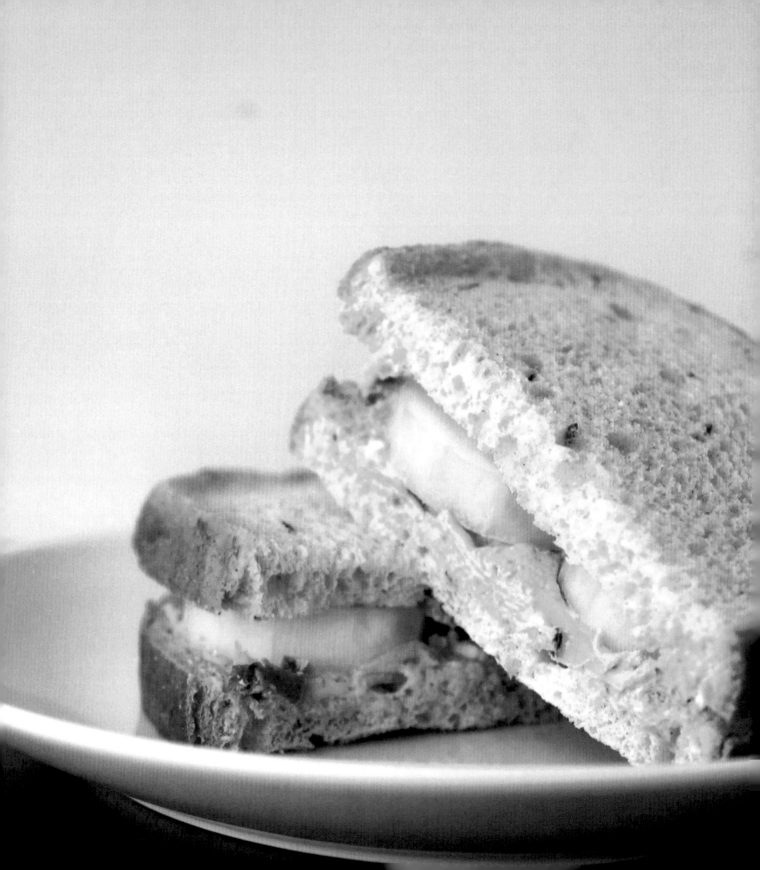

Cucumber Sandwich with Sun Dried Tomato Goat Cheese Spread

Makes 4 sandwiches

2 cucumbers, peeled and sliced

4 oz tube of goat cheese

1 tbsp julienned sun dried tomatoes with oil

1/2 tsp salt

1/4 tsp pepper

1 tbsp soy milk or cow's milk

Russian rye or sourdough bread

Let the goat cheese stand at room temperature for 30 minutes to soften. Combine goat cheese, sun dried tomatoes with oil, salt, pepper and milk in a food processor, then process until smooth.

Spread goat cheese on 4 slices of bread, then add cucumber slices. Top with another slice of bread, cutting crusts off if desired for a more traditional tea sandwich.

Sweet Dill Homemade Refrigerator Pickles

Makes 1 jar of pickles

1 cucumber, peeled and thinly sliced

1 quart sized mason jar

1/4 c. sugar

1 tbsp dried dill

White vinegar

Water

2 tbsp salt

In the mason jar, add sugar, dill and salt. Add 1 c. of vinegar and stir to dissolve sugar. Add cucumber slices, then fill the jar 2/3 up with vinegar. Fill the rest of the jar to a little below the lip with water. Put the lid on and refrigerate for at least 1 week before using. The pickles will stay good for about 2 weeks after that.

Serving suggestions:

-Pickle and cheddar cheese sandwich with a little mustard and mayo

-Great on any burger

-Turkey and pickle sandwich with an herbed mustard plus a little lettuce and tomato is fantastically easy and great for hiking!

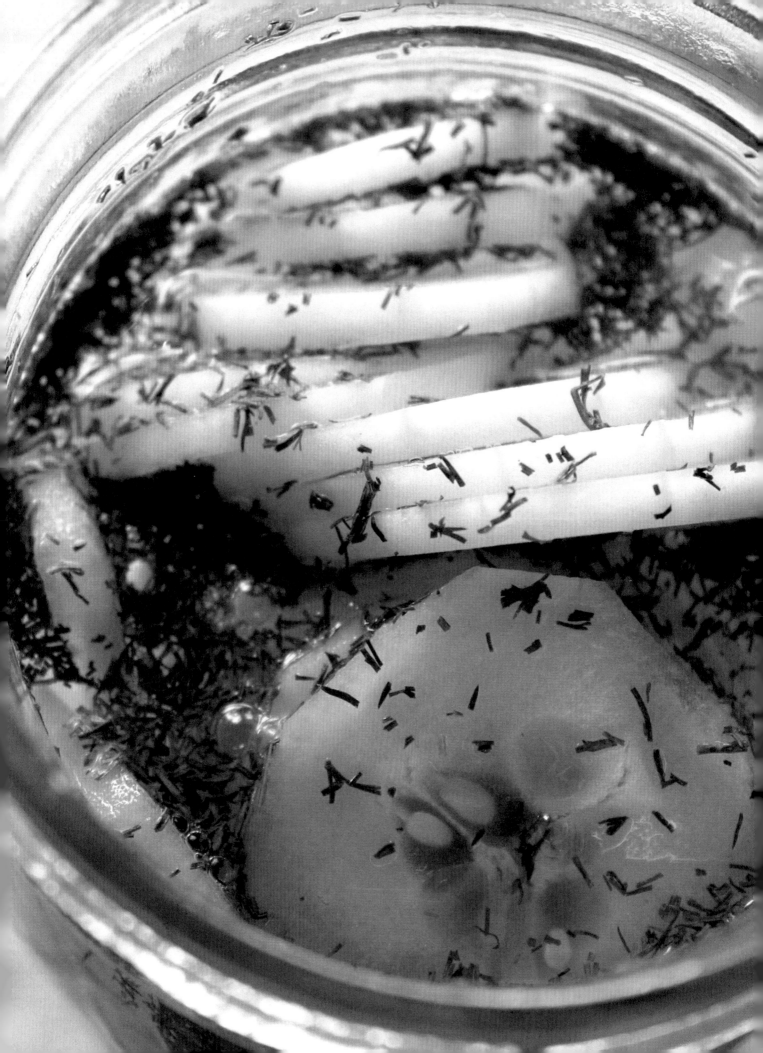

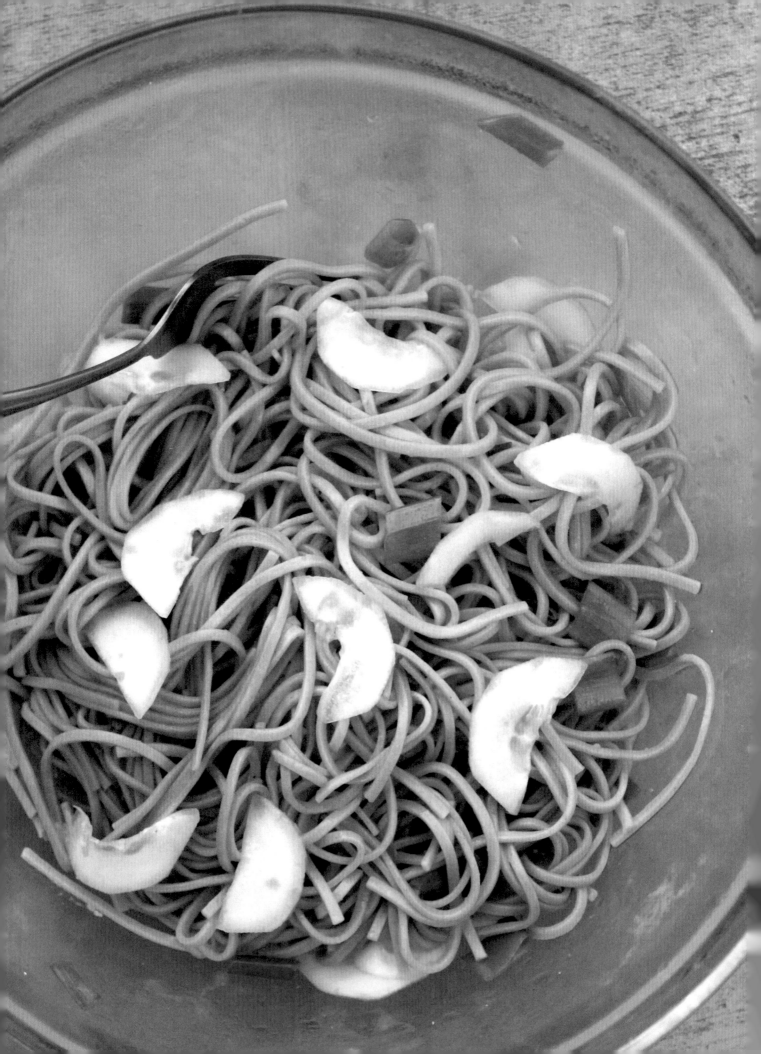

Chilled Soba Noodles with Cucumber

Serves 4

1/2 package soba noodles (or 2 bundles)

1/2 cucumber, peeled, cut into half lengthwise and sliced thinly

Green onions, sliced

Sesame seeds, optional

Dressing:

3 tbsp mirin

4 tbsp rice wine vinegar

1 tbsp sesame oil

1/4 tsp ground ginger

1 tsp sugar

1/4 tsp salt

In a large stock pot, bring water to a boil. Cook soba noodles according to package. Drain and set aside.

Mix together ingredients for dressing in a large bowl. Add noodles, cucumbers and green onion slices. Toss to combine, then cover and chill for at least an hour before serving. Sprinkle sesame seeds over the top just before serving.

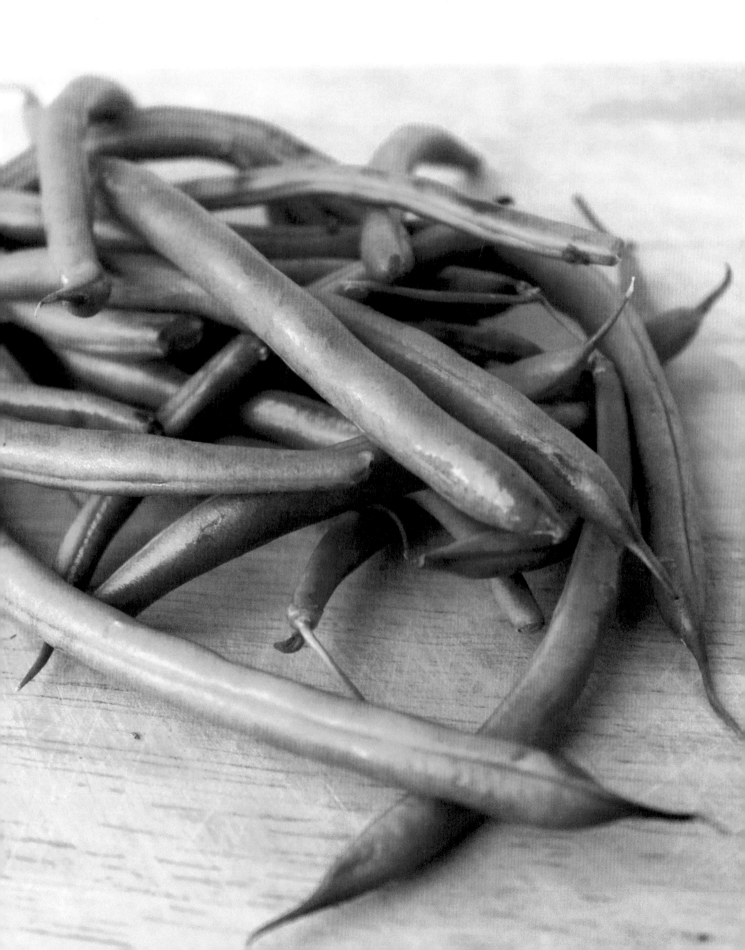

Green Beans

My grandma and I still argue about green beans. Whenever our family gets together, I would always bring beautiful, crisp, barely cooked green beans, which is how I love them. My grandma, on the other hand, loves hers a la cooked to death, as she puts it. Out of a can and boiled to near mush, that's how she has eaten her beans her whole life and no matter how hard I try to convince her that mine are better, she just won't relent. Guess I have to keep trying, huh?

The recipes I have for this section are mainly recreations of staple dishes in my home, especially the spring rolls. I do have to say my new version of spring rolls beats the old, but it's still a close second. These spring rolls are great for a hands-on dinner party where guests can choose what they want in their rolls, but they also make a great ahead of time appetizer. Either way, they are delicious.

Green Bean Spring Rolls

Makes about 1 dozen rolls

2 chicken breasts, cut into 3 piece each and pounded to 1/2" thick

¼ c. ponzu

2 tbsp mirin

1 tsp grated ginger

1 glove garlic, minced

½ c. water

1 package shredded carrots

½ c. rice vinegar

1 tbsp sugar

1 bunch green onions, sliced

1 lb. green beans

1 package bean threads

Mint leaves

Cilantro leaves

Rice paper

Dressing:

1/4 c. peanut butter, chunky preferred

1/4 c. soy sauce

2 tbsp rice vinegar

1 tbsp mirin

To cook chicken, add ponzu, mirin, ginger, garlic and water in a large sauté pan. Bring to a boil, then reduce to a gentle simmer. Add chicken and gently poach for 7-8 minutes, turning once. Remove chicken from pan and set aside to cool. Cut into thin strips when able to be handled.

For marinated carrots, mix together carrots, vinegar, green onions and sugar, then set aside to marinate.

Bring a large pot of water to a boil, then add green beans. Cook for 1 minute, then remove and place beans into an ice water bath to stop them from cooking. Once chilled, drain and set aside.

Place bean threads in a shallow baking dish, then top with boiling water. Let soak for 5-6 minutes, or until soft. Drain and set aside.

To assemble rolls, fill a glass pie plate with warm water. Dip a rice paper sheet into the water and let soak until just malleable, but not so soft that they tear. Remove paper from water and place on a cutting board or plate. Tear a small handful of bean threads, then place on rice paper. Top with a few chicken slices, some marinated carrots, a couple of green beans, a mint leaf, and a cilantro leaf. Carefully roll up the paper without tearing it (it will take a few practice ones to learn the technique), then tuck the ends under and set aside on a plate. Repeat until you run out of ingredients.

For dipping sauce, mix together all ingredients until smooth and slightly runny. Add water if needed to make sauce thinner. Serve with the spring rolls.

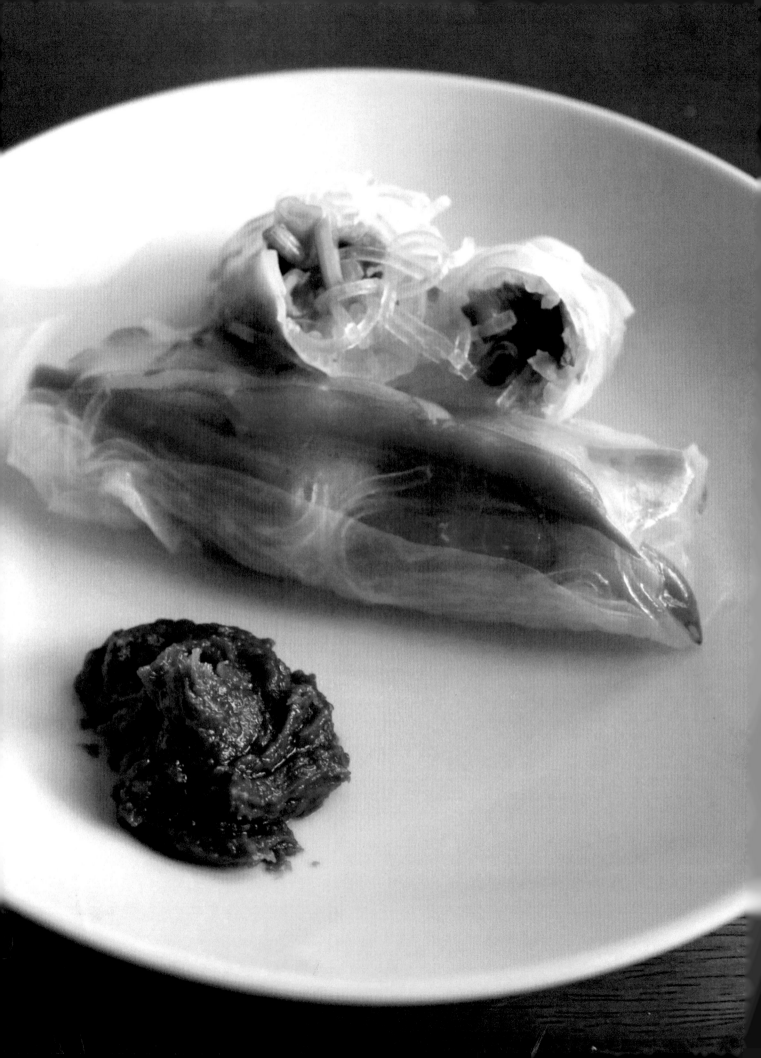

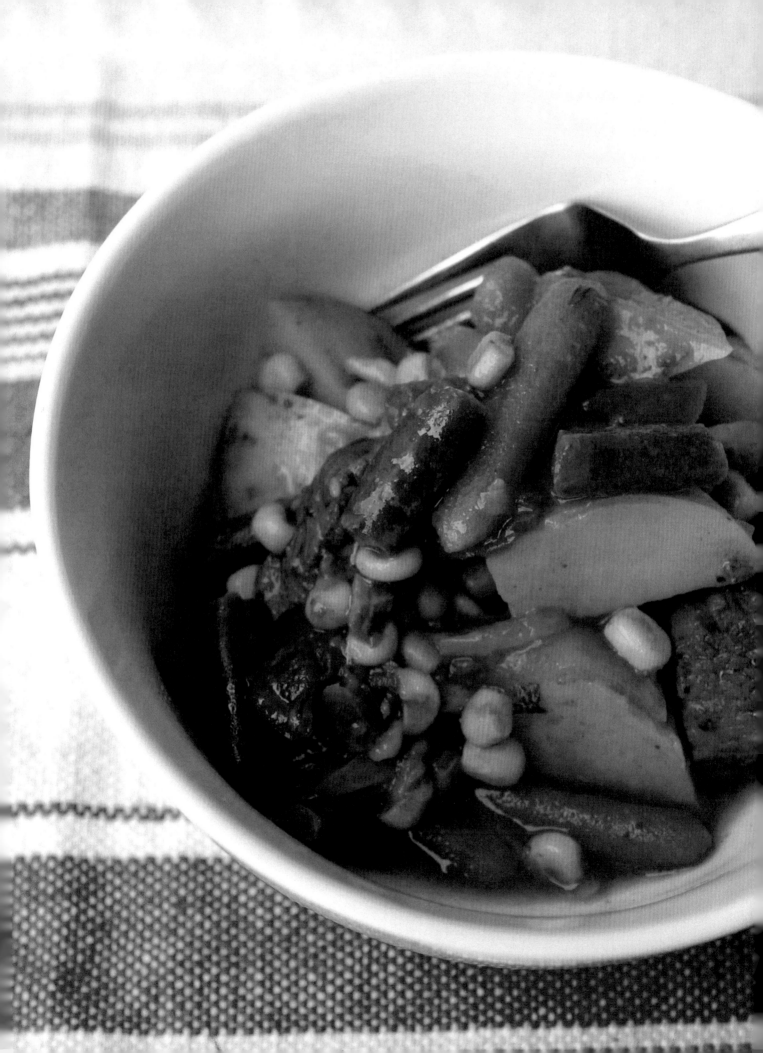

Beef Stew with Green Beans

Serves 4

¾ lb. sirloin steak, cubed

1 onion, chopped

2 cloves garlic, minced

2 tbsp AP flour

2 Yukon Gold potatoes, cubed

2 tomatoes, cut into wedges

1 c. baby carrots

3 c. beef broth

1 c. red wine

1 tbsp dried parsley

1 tsp dried thyme

1 tbsp salt

1 tsp pepper

1 c. green beans, thawed if frozen

1 c. corn, thawed if frozen

In a Dutch oven over medium-high heat, add 1 tbsp olive oil, then cook onion and garlic for 2 minutes, until onion begins to brown. Remove onion from pan, then add beef cubes. Brown beef, turning every minute or so to brown on all side. Sprinkle flour over beef, cook for 30 more seconds, then add all remaining ingredients except green beans and corn.

Bring to a boil, then reduce to simmer and cook for 45 minutes, or until potatoes and carrots are cooked. Add green beans and corn and cook for another 5 minutes. Serve hot with crunchy bread.

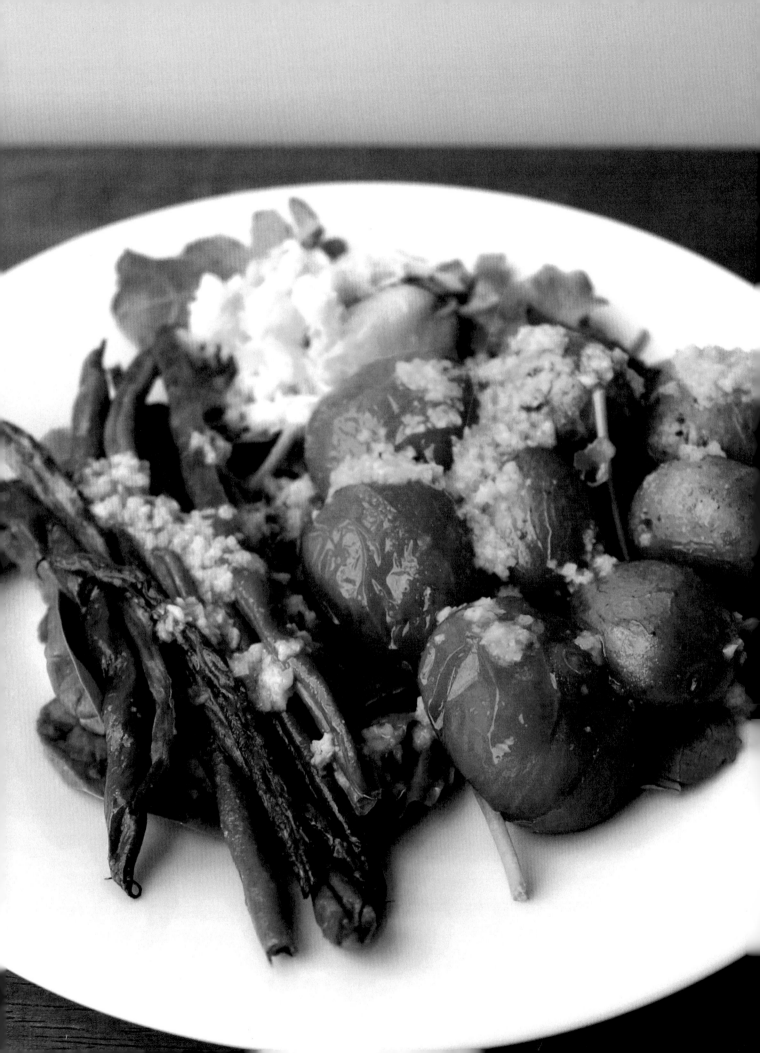

Roasted Veggie Salad with Crab

Serves 2

1/2 lb green beans, trimmed

6 small tomatoes

8 baby red potatoes

1/4 lb crab

1 c. greens

Dressing:

1 tbsp champagne or white wine vinegar

3 tbsp olive oil

5 roasted garlic cloves

1/4 tsp salt

1/8 tsp pepper

Heat oven to 400 F. Put beans, tomatoes and potatoes in a medium ceramic or glass baking dish, then toss with olive oil, salt and pepper. Roast in oven for 20-25 minutes, taking beans out after 15. Set aside.

For dressing, combine all ingredients in a food processor and process until smooth. To make salad, lay half of the greens on each plate, then top with beans, tomatoes and potatoes. Add crab to each plate, then drizzle with dressing.

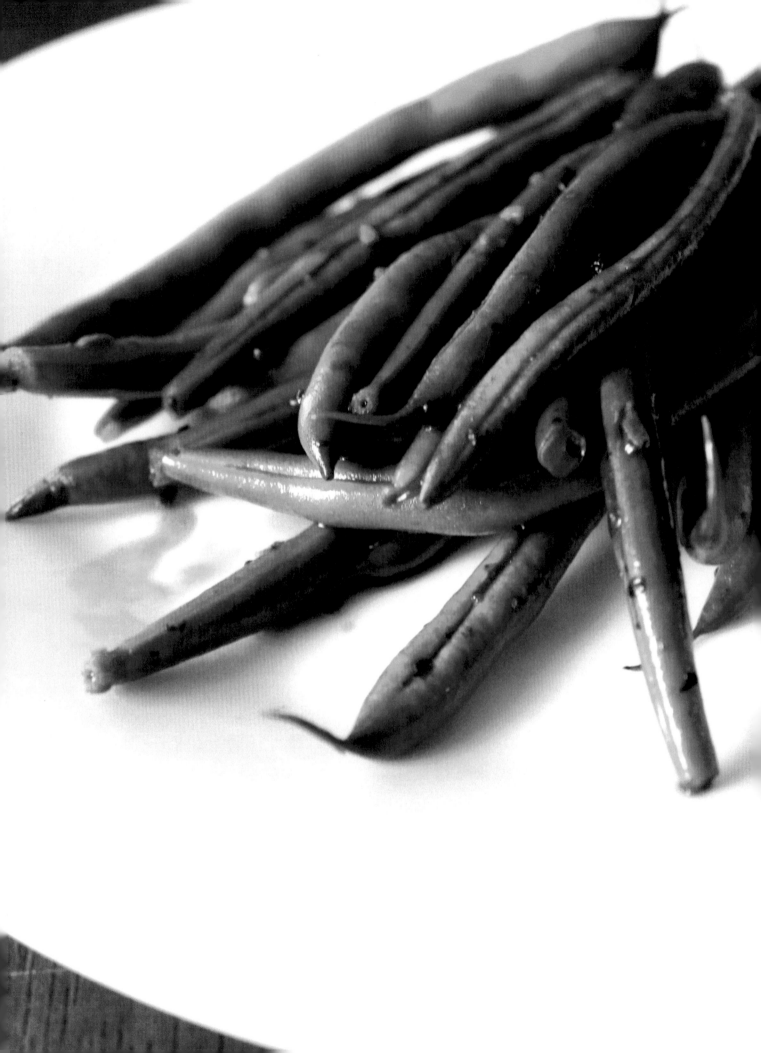

Green Beans in a Garlic Black Bean Sauce

Serves 4

1 lb. green beans, ends trimmed

2 tbsp garlic black bean sauce (found in Asian section of store)

2 tbsp mirin

Combine garlic black bean sauce and mirin in a large sauté pan and set aside. Bring a large stockpot of water to a boil. Add green beans and cook for 1 minute. Remove green beans and place into sauté pan, along with 1/2 c. water. Put sauté pan on the burner used for the boiling water and cook over medium high heat for 1 minute, tossing beans into sauce. Place beans on a platter, then spoon sauce over and serve.

Risotto with Garlicky Green Beans and Shrimp

Serves 4

1 lb green beans, trimmed and cut into half

1 small onion, diced

4 cloves garlic, minced

2 tbsp olive oil

1 c. Arborio rice

About 3 cups chicken or vegetable stock

1/2 c. wine

1/2 tsp salt

1/4 tsp pepper

1 tbsp olive oil

3/4 lb shrimp, peeled, deveined and patted dry

In a large stock pot, bring an inch of water to a boil. Add green beans and cook for 1 minute, then drain and set aside.

Heat a medium saucepan over medium heat. Add 1 tbsp oil and onions, and sauté for 2-3 minutes or until they begin to get translucent but not brown. Add the other tbsp. of oil and 1/2 of the garlic, cook for another minute. Stir in rice until the rice is coated with oil. Combine wine and chicken stock, then add about 1 c. of liquid to the rice. Bring to a simmer, and let cook until the liquid is absorbed. Add another 1 c. of liquid and repeat. Stir every few minutes to prevent rice from sticking to the bottom of the pan.

For the last 1/2 cup of liquid, turn off heat and cover. Let rice continue to cook off heat while the shrimp are cooking.

Heat a large sauté pan over medium high heat. Add 1 tbsp oil, then cook shrimp until just pink. Add garlic and green beans and cook for another minute, tossing to combine. Sprinkle with salt and pepper and serve shrimp mixture over risotto.

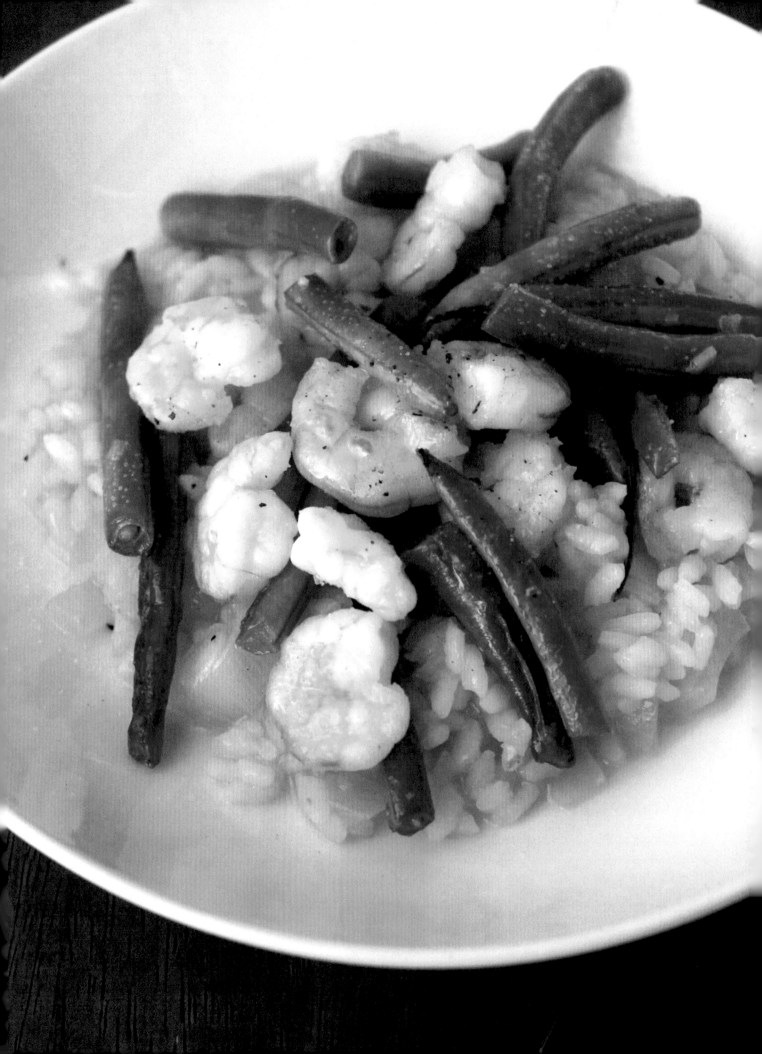

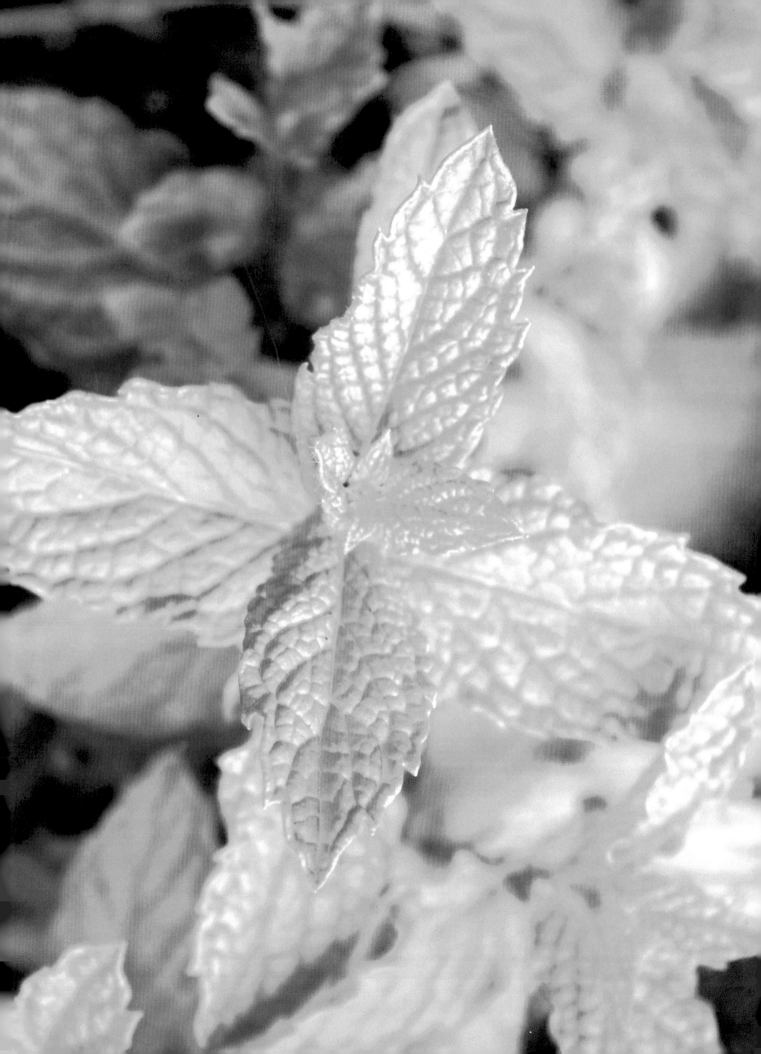

Lettuce

Oh lettuce. That plain vegetable that usually gets drowned in dressing to hide the fact that its, well, kind of plain. But lettuce doesn't have to be only in a salad! It makes a great wrapper, as in my hoisin chicken lettuce wraps, which I have been making since college.

Lettuce is also great when grilled. I never even heard of grilling lettuce until a former co-worker mentioned that he would always grill his lettuce and arugula. Once I tried it, I became hooked!

And of course, lettuce makes a great salad base, in which I've included 3 of my favorites. But don't make me choose between them, because I definitely cannot!

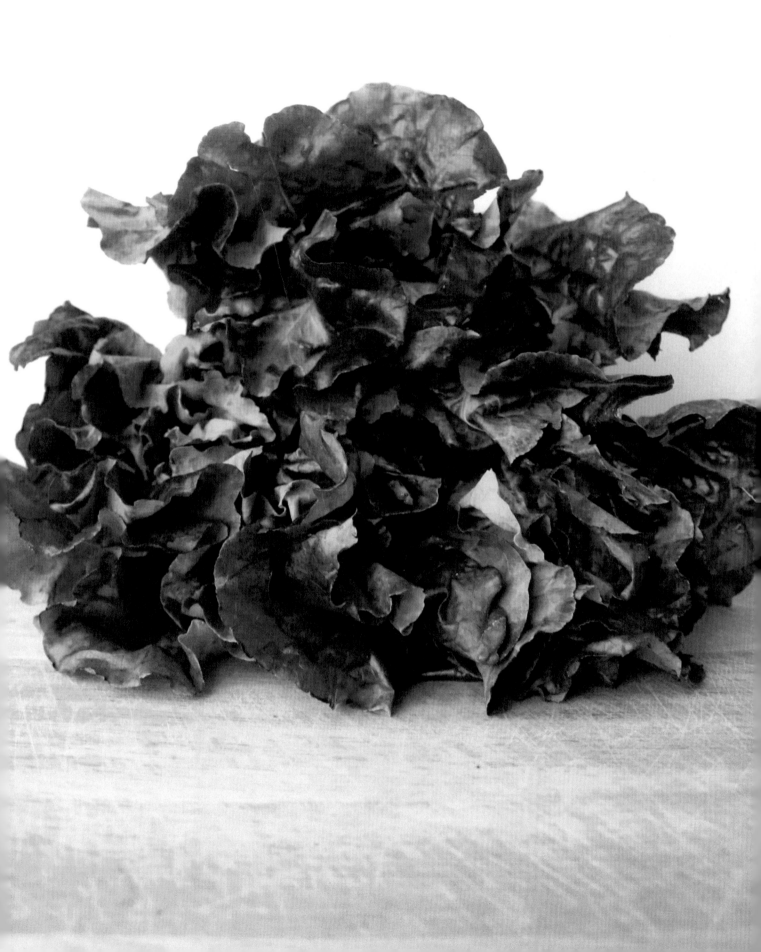

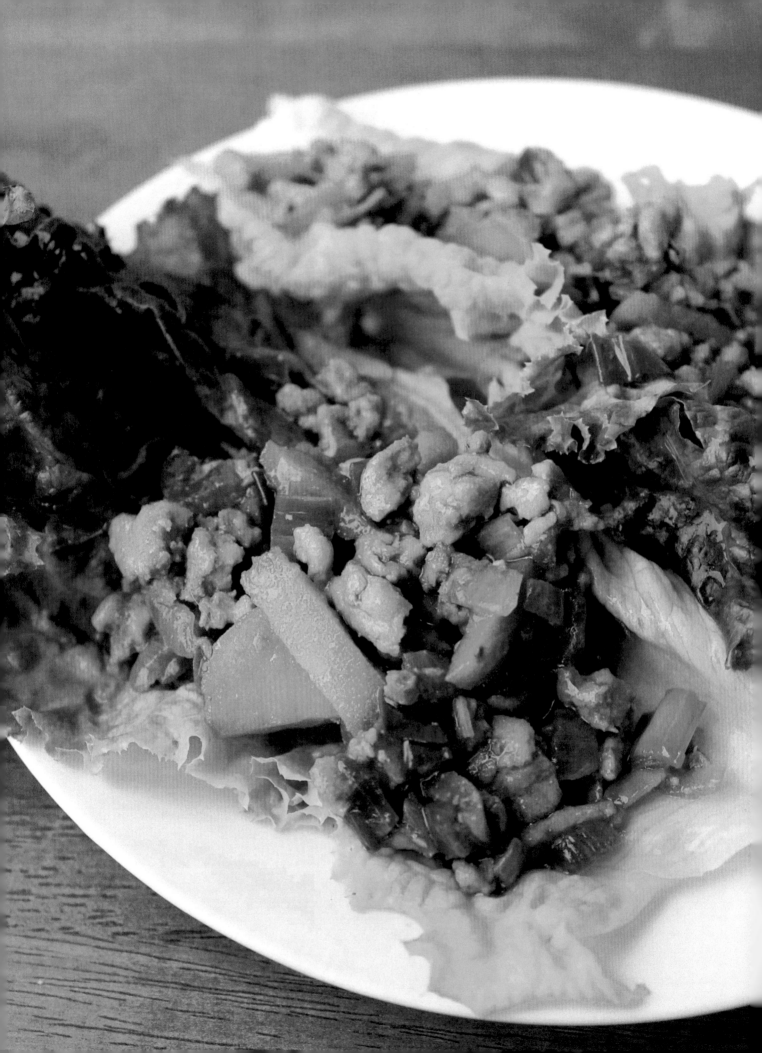

Hoisin Chicken Lettuce Wraps

Serves 4

1 lb ground chicken

½ onion, diced

2 garlic cloves, minced

1 can water chestnuts, drained and chopped

¼ c. soy sauce

¼ c. hoisin

1 tbsp sesame oil

2 green onions, sliced

Red leaf lettuce, rinsed, leaves separated individually

In a large sauté pan, heat 1 tbsp olive oil over medium-high heat. Add onions and garlic, and sauté for 2 minutes until onion begins to get translucent. Add chicken and brown, about 4-5 minutes, stirring occasionally until no more pink remains.

Add water chestnuts, soy sauce, hoisin, sesame oil, and green onions. Stir to combine.

To serve, pour chicken mixture into a large bowl and let people grab their own lettuce leaves and spoon the chicken mixture into the leaves. Roll up the leaves and devour.

Summer Simple Salad

Serves 4

1 head lettuce, rinsed and chopped into large pieces

4 tomatoes, chopped

2 c. croutons

Dressing:

2 tbsp balsamic vinegar

6 tbsp olive oil

1 tsp salt

½ tsp pepper

In 4 separate bowls, divide lettuce pieces. Top each with some tomato and croutons. Whisk together ingredients for dressing, then pour a little on top of each salad. Toss to coat, then serve.

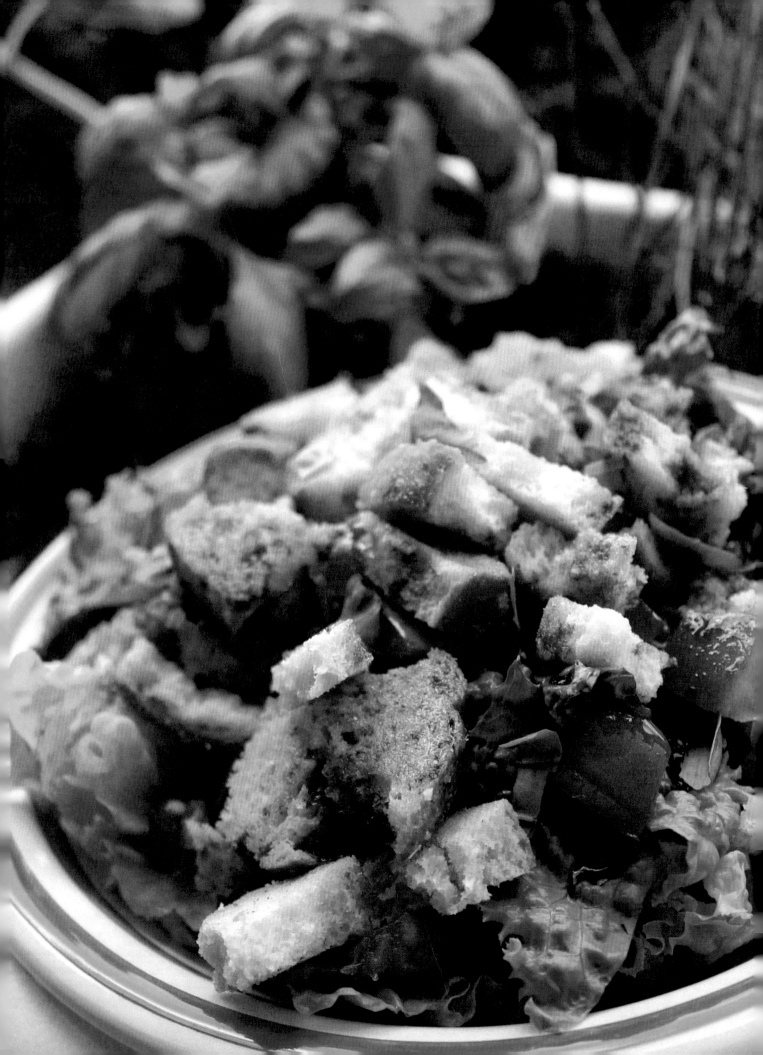

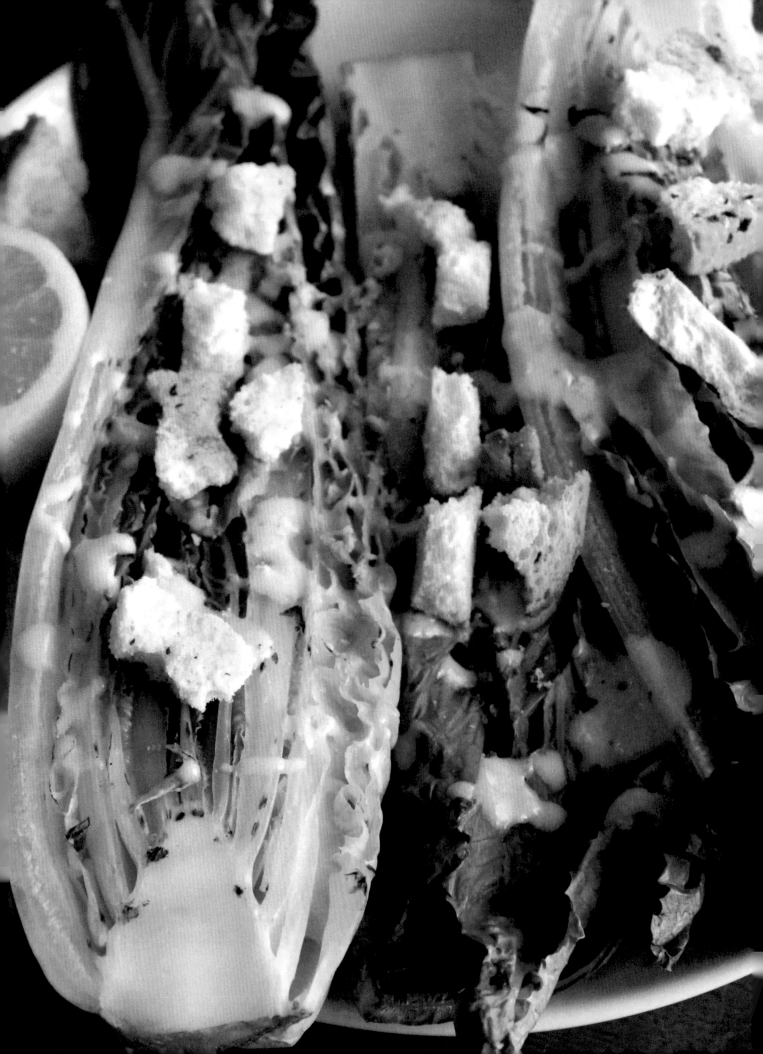

Grilled Romaine Caesar Salad

Serves 6

3 hearts of Romaine, cut in half lengthwise

Croutons

Lemon slices

Dressing:

2 tbsp vegan mayo

6 tbsp oil

6 tbsp lemon juice

4 cloves garlic

2 tbsp Dijon mustard

4 dashes Worcestershire sauce

1/4 tsp salt

1/4 tsp pepper

To make dressing, combine all ingredients in a food processor and process until smooth. Set aside.

Heat a grill pan or grill over medium high heat. Lay romaine heart halves cut side down on grill. Grill for 1 minute or until grill marks begin to appear on the lettuce. Remove and set on a large platter with grill side up.

Sprinkle croutons over the top, then drizzle with dressing. Place lemon slices around lettuce as a garnish and serve.

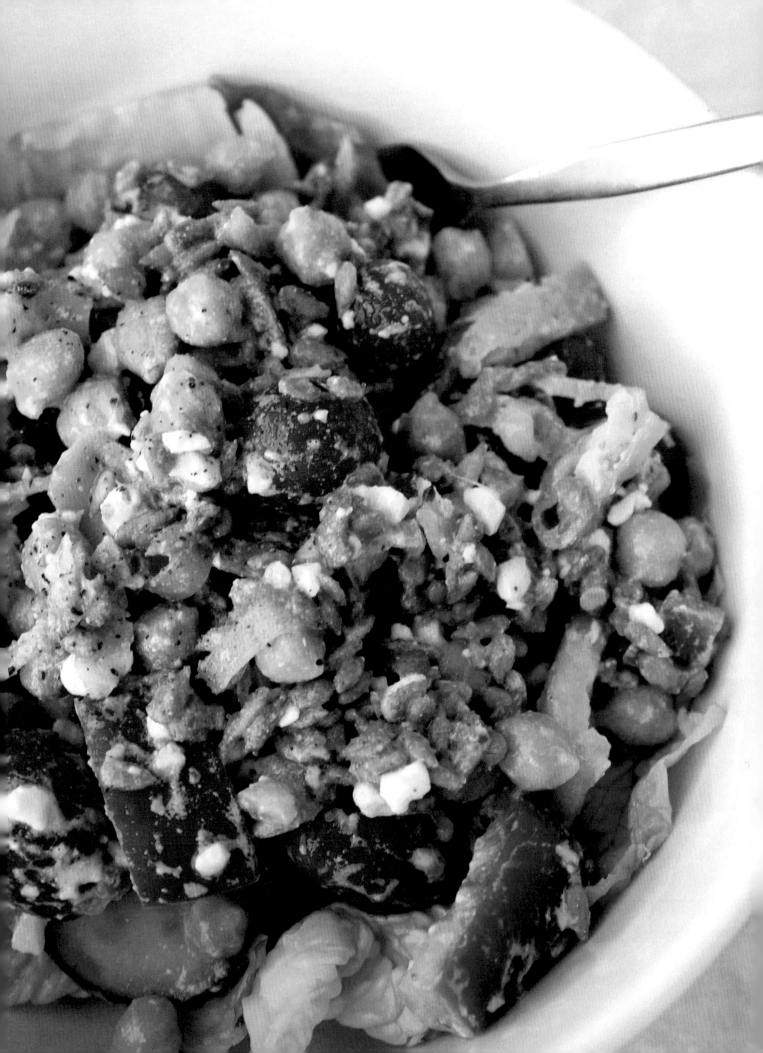

Greek Salad over Romaine

Serves 4

Romaine lettuce, chopped

1 pint grape tomatoes

1 yellow bell pepper, chopped

1/2 cucumber, sliced

2 tbsp pepperoncinis

2 tbsp sunflower seeds

1 can chickpeas, drained and rinsed

Dressing:

1/3 c. olive oil

2 tbsp lemon juice

1/4 tsp dried oregano

1/4 tsp salt

1/8 tsp pepper

2 tbsp feta, crumbled

In a large bowl, layer lettuce, tomatoes, bell pepper, cucumber, chickpeas and pepperoncinis. Sprinkle over sesame seeds.

For the dressing, combine all ingredients and stir to mix, leaving chunks of feta cheese. Pour over veggies and toss to combine.

Grilled Steak Salad with Corn

Makes 4 salads

2 sirloin steaks, top loin

1/4 tsp each coriander, chili powder, cumin, paprika, salt, pepper

2 c. corn

1/2 c. halved grape tomatoes

Romaine lettuce, chopped

Dressing:

Juice of 1 lime

1/2 c. olive oil

1 tsp pomegranate molasses or sugar

1/2 tsp Mexican hot sauce

1 handful cilantro, chopped

1/4 tsp salt

1/8 tsp pepper

In a medium bowl, combine all ingredients for the dressing. Add corn and tomato halves, and set aside to marinate. For the steaks, mix together spices, then rub half on each steak. Let stand for 10 minutes, then grill over medium-high heat until medium rare, flipping once. Remove from pan and let rest for 10 minutes. Slice thinly.

Put a few handfuls of lettuce into each bowl, then top with some steak slices and a spoonful or two of the corn mixture.

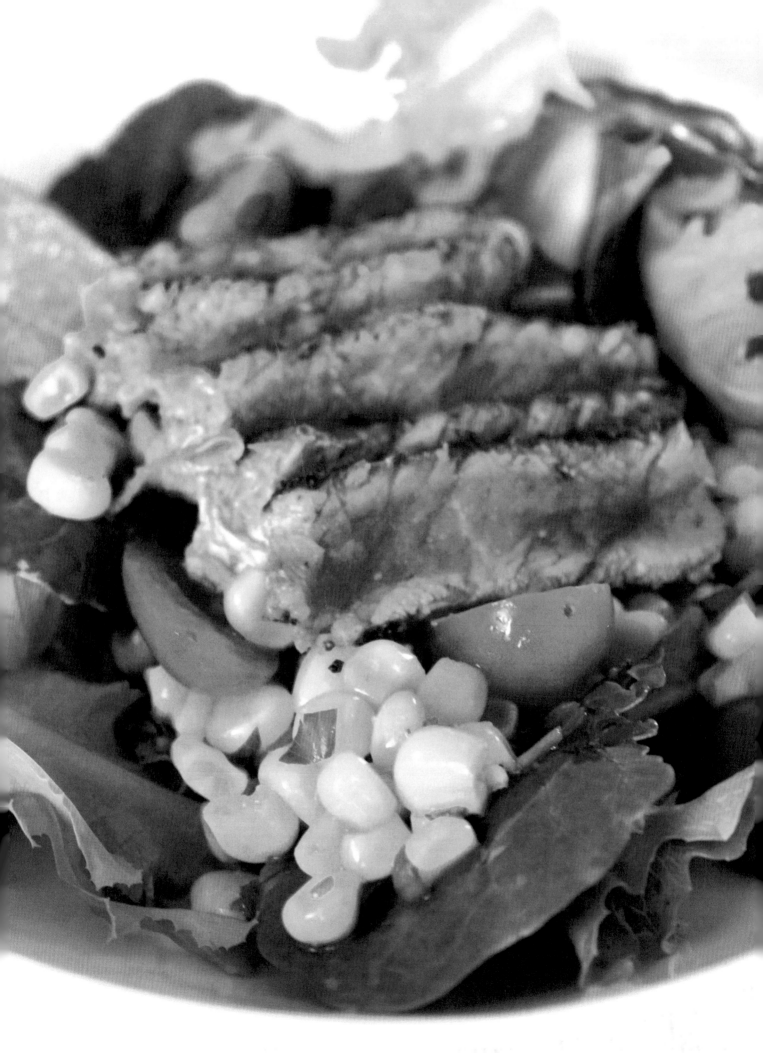

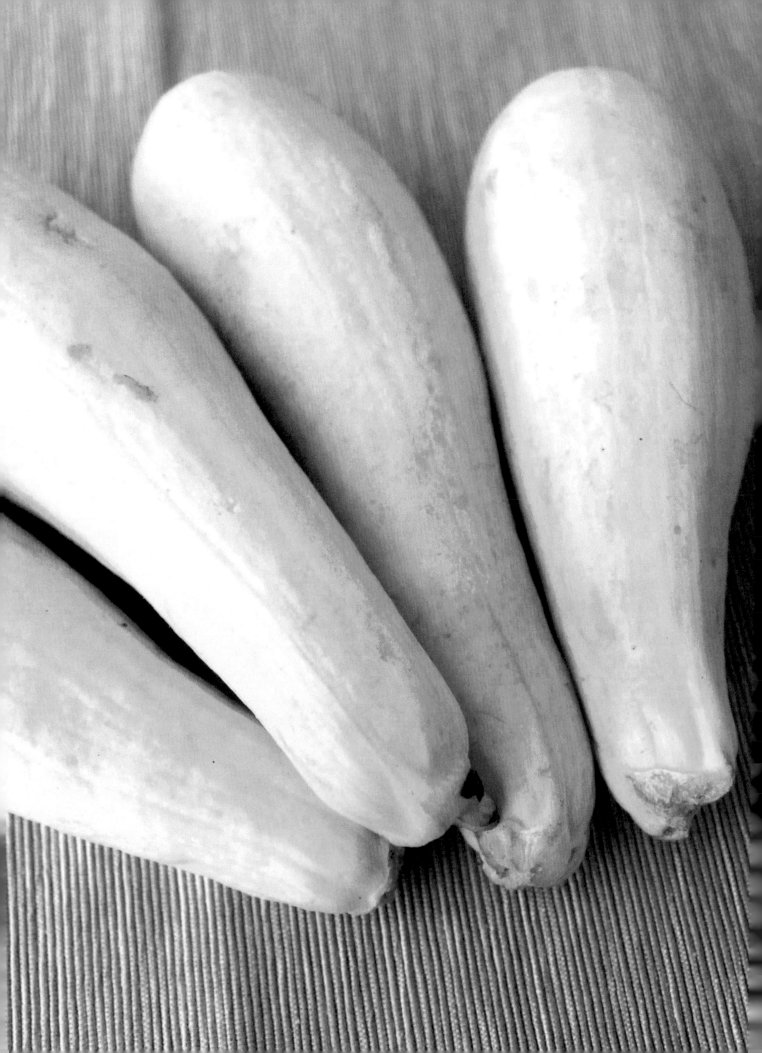

Summer Squash

I never heard of summer squash until I started collecting cookbooks. I remember the recipe was a risotto with summer squash. I'd heard of zucchini, which is related, but never summer squash. And now, I love summer squash!

Summer squash is a general term for thin skinned immature squash that peaks in, well, summer. In my recipes, I used all yellow summer squash, which is typically differentiated from zucchini, even though it's also a summer squash, but it's so well known by its own name that it gets its own chapter.

The two most popular yellow summer squashes are crookneck and pattypan. I prefer the crookneck, just because it's easier to cut up, in my opinion, but any summer squash will do in these recipes, even zucchini.

The best summer squash recipe from this book has got to be the sandwich. Oh my goodness it was delicious, and did I mention really easy to make? It's just grilled chicken and veggies with some honey BBQ sauce. I think I need to make another one soon.

Summer Squash and Parmesan on Crostini

Makes about 12 appetizers

2 summer squash, diced

2 cloves garlic, minced

10 fennel seeds

1/4 tsp coriander

1/4 tsp salt

1/8 tsp pepper

2 tbsp grated parmesan or pecorino romano

Store brought crostinis, or toasted baguette slices

In a sauté pan, heat 1 tbsp oil over medium high heat. Cook garlic and fennel seeds for 30 seconds, then add squash, salt and pepper. Cook squash for 5 minutes, tossing every minute or so, until cooked through but not mushy. Sprinkle with coriander and toss to combine.

Lay 12 crostinis on a platter, and add a spoonful of squash on top of each. Sprinkle with grated parmesan and serve.

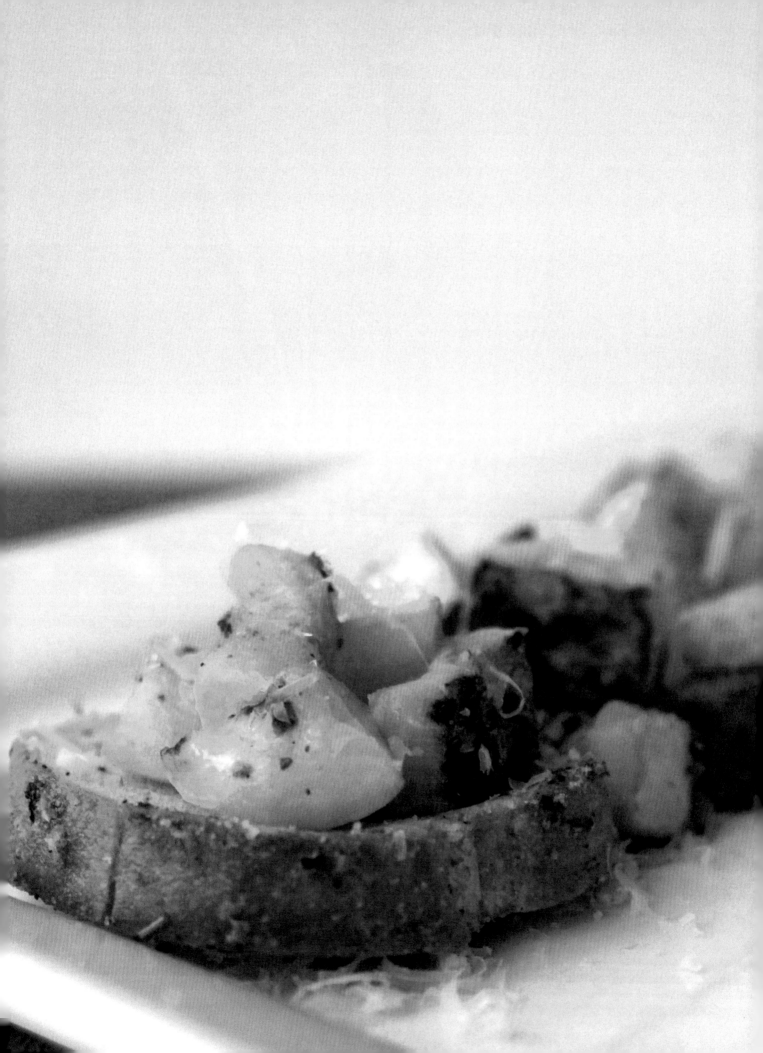

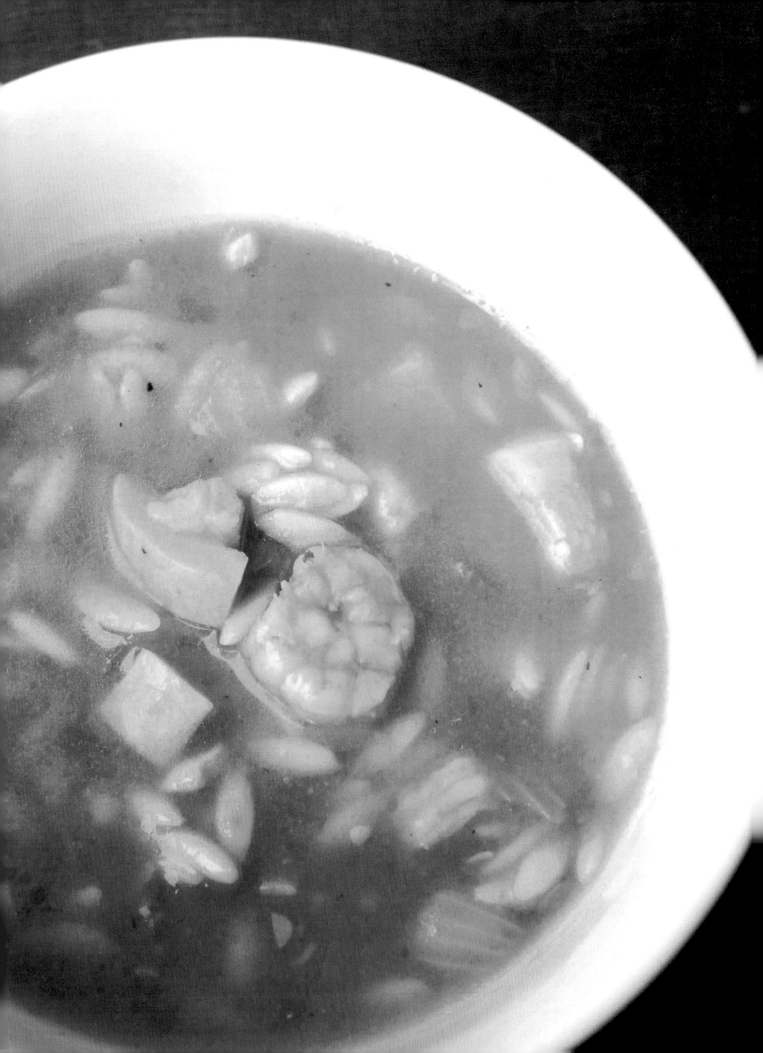

Summer Squash and Shrimp Soup with Orzo

Serves 4

2 summer squash, cubed

½ lb. medium shrimp, peeled and deveined

½ onion, diced

2 cloves garlic, minced

4 c. vegetable stock

½ c. orzo

2 tsp salt

½ tsp pepper

In a large stock pot, heat 1 tbsp oil over medium heat. Add onion and garlic and sauté for 3 minutes, or until onion becomes translucent. Add summer squash and cook for another 2 minutes. Add all remaining ingredients, then bring to a boil. Reduce to low and simmer for 8 minutes, until orzo is cooked. Serve hot.

Grilled Summer Squash and Chicken Sandwich with Honey BBQ Sauce

Makes 4 sandwiches

2 summer squash, sliced thinly into coins using a mandolin

1 sweet onion, cut in half and sliced

1 red sweet pepper, cut into strips

2 chicken breasts

4 ciabatta, cut in half

1/2 c. honey BBQ sauce, heated

For the chicken, cut each chicken breast in half, then pound to 1/2" thick. Season with salt and pepper. Heat a grill pan or electric grill over medium high heat, and cook chicken until done, about 2-3 minutes per side. Remove from heat and set aside, keeping warm.

Toss onion and peppers in 1 tbsp olive oil, 1/2 tsp salt and 1/4 tsp pepper. Toss the squash in a separate bowl with 1 tsp olive oil, 1/4 tsp salt and 1/8 tsp pepper. Grill for about 10 minutes total, adding squash after the first five minutes. The onions and squash should be soft while the peppers will still be crisp tender.

Cut the cooked chicken into strips, then toss with BBQ sauce. Divide chicken between ciabattas, then top each with squash mixture. Drizzle a little more BBQ sauce on top, then top with other half of ciabatta. Serve cut in half diagonally.

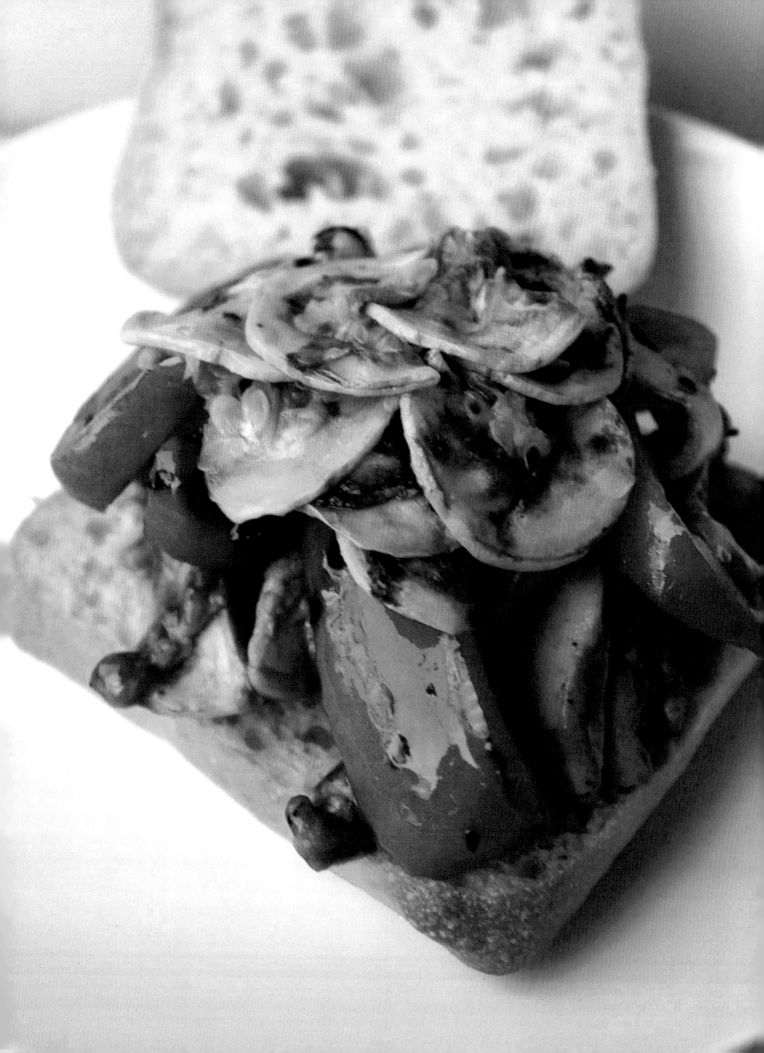

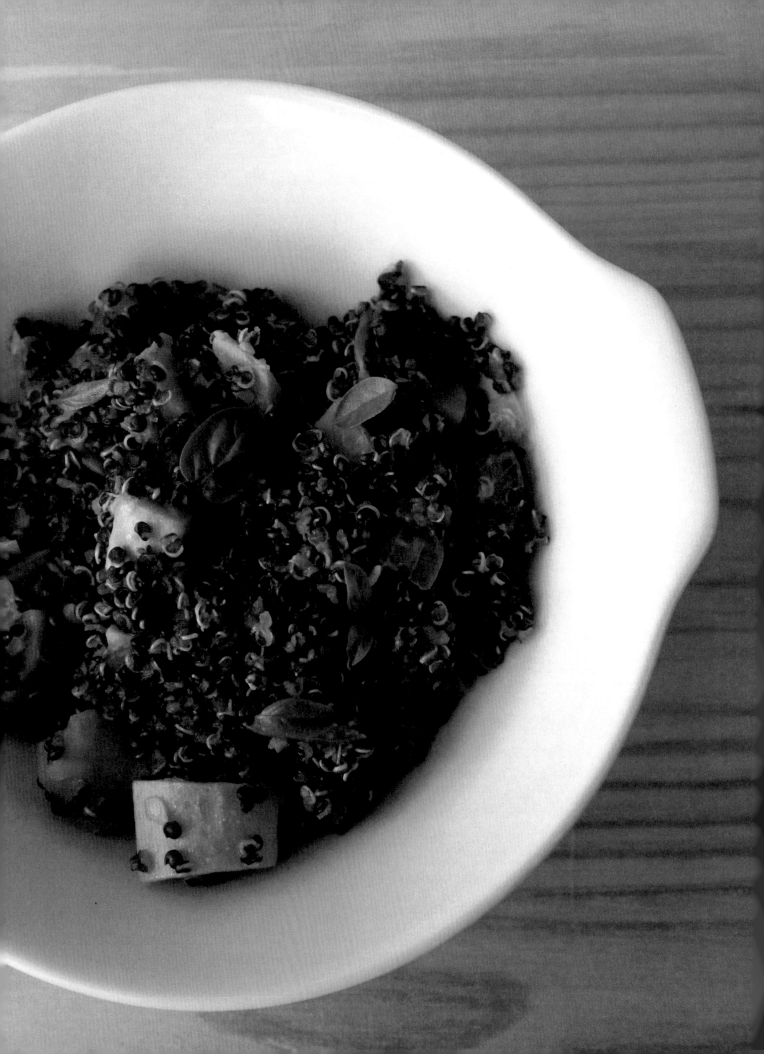

Summer Squash and Quinoa Pilaf

Serves 4

1/2 small onion, diced

1 clove garlic, minced

2 summer squash, diced

1/2 tsp salt

1/4 tsp pepper

1 tsp dried parsley

1 c. red or white quinoa, rinsed

1 3/4 c. chicken or vegetable stock

Basil, for garnish

In a medium saucepan, heat 1 tbsp oil over medium heat. Add onions, and sauté for 3 minutes or until onions begin to get translucent. Add garlic and summer squash, and sauté for 1 minute. Add quinoa, and sauté for 1 additional minute. Pour in stock, along with salt, pepper and parsley. Bring to a boil, then reduce to a simmer and cook for 18-20 minutes, or until almost all the liquid is absorbed. Set aside for 5 minutes to let the rest of the liquid absorb, then serve with basil leaves on top for garnish.

Summer Squash Burger

Serves 4

1 lb. ground beef

3 tbsp julienned sun dried tomatoes, with oil

2 summer squash, sliced thinly

1 sweet onion, sliced thinly

1 clove garlic, minced

Lettuce

Hamburger buns

Ketchup, mustard, mayo

In a large bowl, combine ground beef and sun dried tomatoes, sprinkling with 1/2 tsp salt and 1/4 tsp pepper. Using your hands, mush the tomatoes into the beef until well blended. Divide into fourths and then shape each fourth into a patty, making a slight dent in the middle with your thumb.

Heat a grill or grill pan over medium high heat. Cook burger patties to desired doneness.

Meanwhile, heat a large sauté pan over medium heat. Add onions and sauté until golden brown, about 10 minutes. Add garlic and sauté for 1 minute. Remove onions and set aside. Add half of the summer squash and sauté until cooked and barely translucent, about 6-7 minutes. Set aside with the onions, then cook the other half of the squash.

To assemble burgers, put a burger patty on the bottom of each bun, then top with onions, summer squash slices and some pieces of lettuce. Add condiments, if desired, and serve with a cold beer.

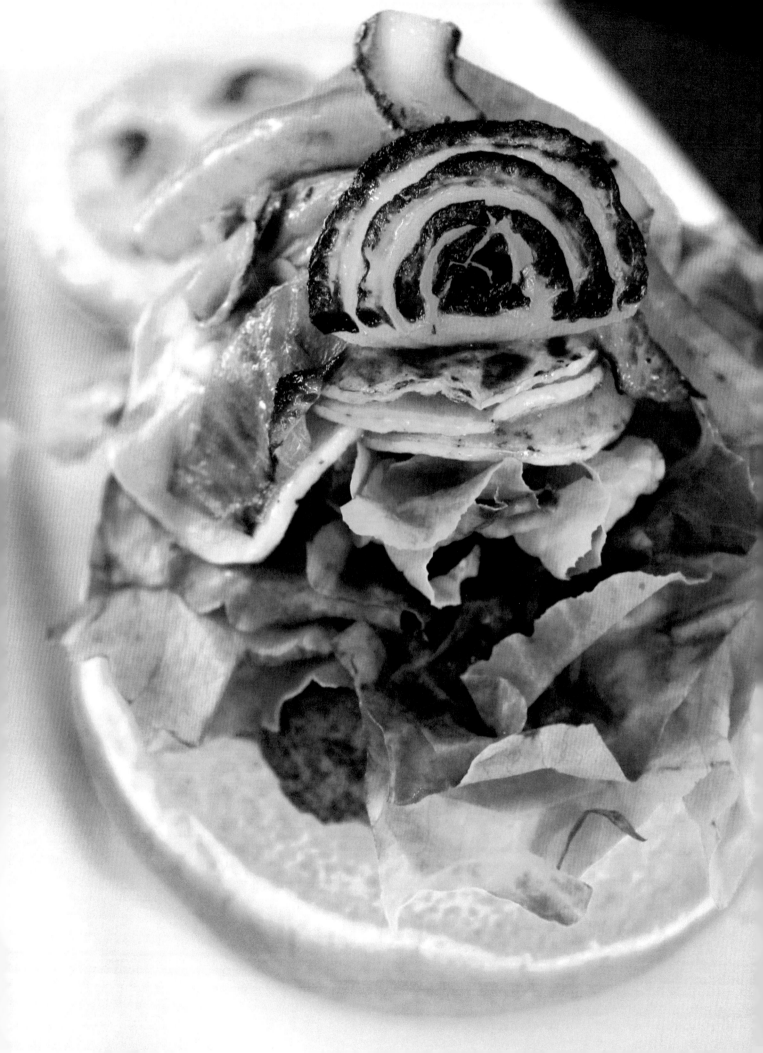

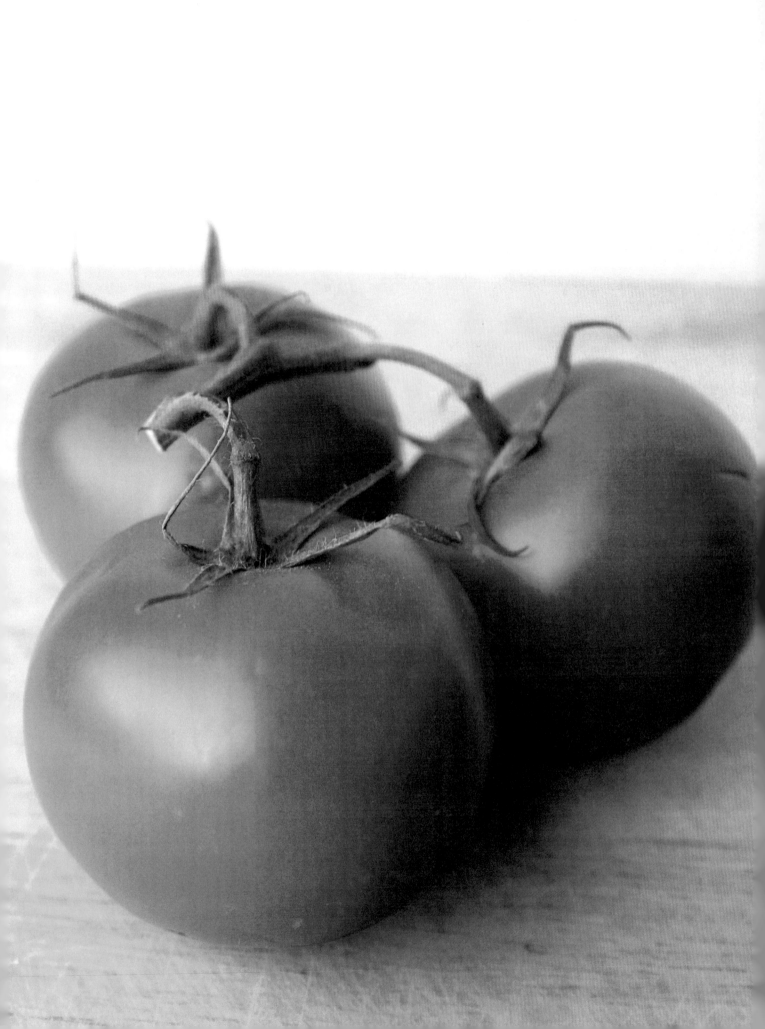

Tomatoes

Tomatoes and corn are the ultimate summer veggies. Tomatoes in the salad, corn on the grill. That's how my family did summer barbecues. But tomatoes shouldn't be just in a salad, especially when they are at their peak.

Tomatoes now come in every shape, size and color at the store, from tiny cherry tomatoes to huge beefsteak heirlooms. All are delicious and perfect for savoring.

I've always been a sucker for a good BLT, but my BKTAC (bacon, kale, tomato, avocado and crab) sandwich hits it out of the park. The crab and bacon pair so well together, and the creamy avocado balances the salt. Grab the ingredients and whip up a sandwich tonight!

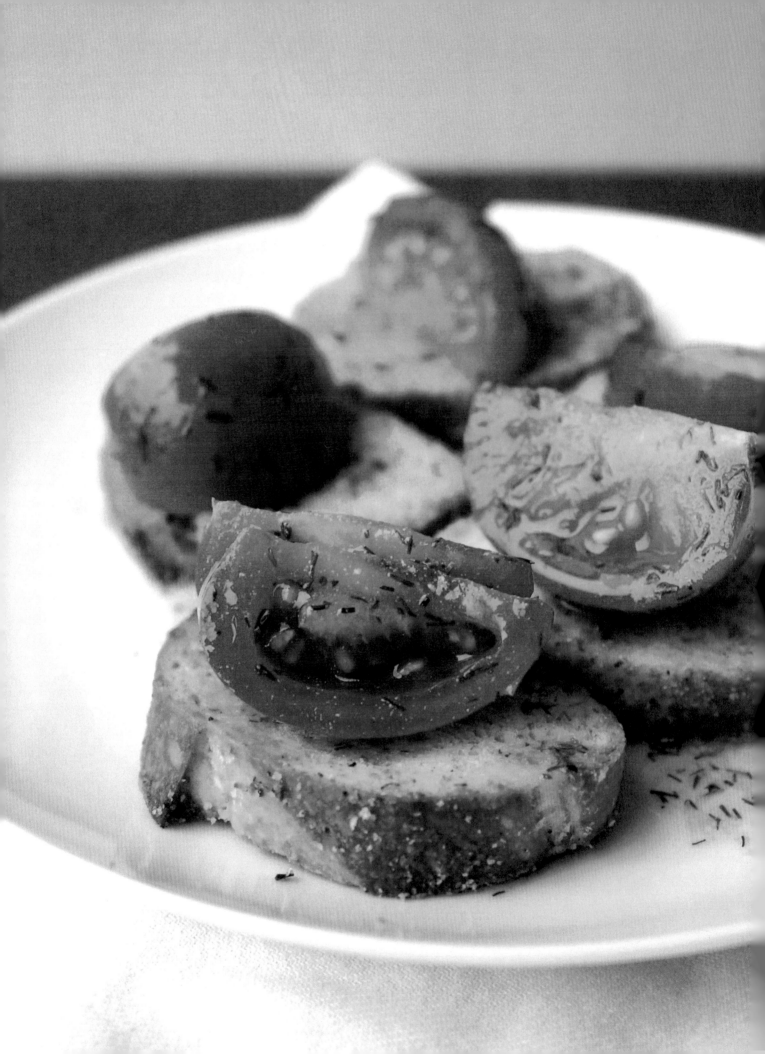

Marinated Dill Mustard Tomatoes on Crostini

Serves 4

1 lb cocktail or grape tomatoes, cut into wedges or in half

1/4 c. olive oil

1/4 c. red wine vinegar

1 tsp dry mustard

1 tsp dill

1/4 tsp salt

1/8 tsp pepper

Crostinis or oven toasted baguettes

Mix all ingredients except crostinis in a large bowl. Stir to combine, and let marinate at room temperature for 30 minutes or in the fridge for 2 hours. If chilled, let come to room temp before serving.

Put a spoonful of tomatoes on each crostini, then drizzle marinade over. Eat immediately.

Creamy Dairy-Free Tomato Soup

Serves 4

4 medium tomatoes, seeded and diced

1/2 large onion, diced

2 garlic cloves, minced

2 tsp tomato paste

4 c. chicken or vegetable stock

1 tsp salt

1/2 tsp pepper

1 can red kidney beans, drained and rinsed

In a large stock pot, heat 1 tbsp oil over medium heat. Add onions and sauté until translucent, about 5 minutes. Add garlic and tomatoes and sauté for 5 more minutes or until tomatoes release their juices. Add remaining ingredients and bring to a boil. Reduce to a simmer and cook for 10 minutes, covered. Set aside to cool, then add kidney beans.

Pour soup into a blender and blend until smooth. For a chunkier soup, use an immersion blender. Serve hot with crusty bread.

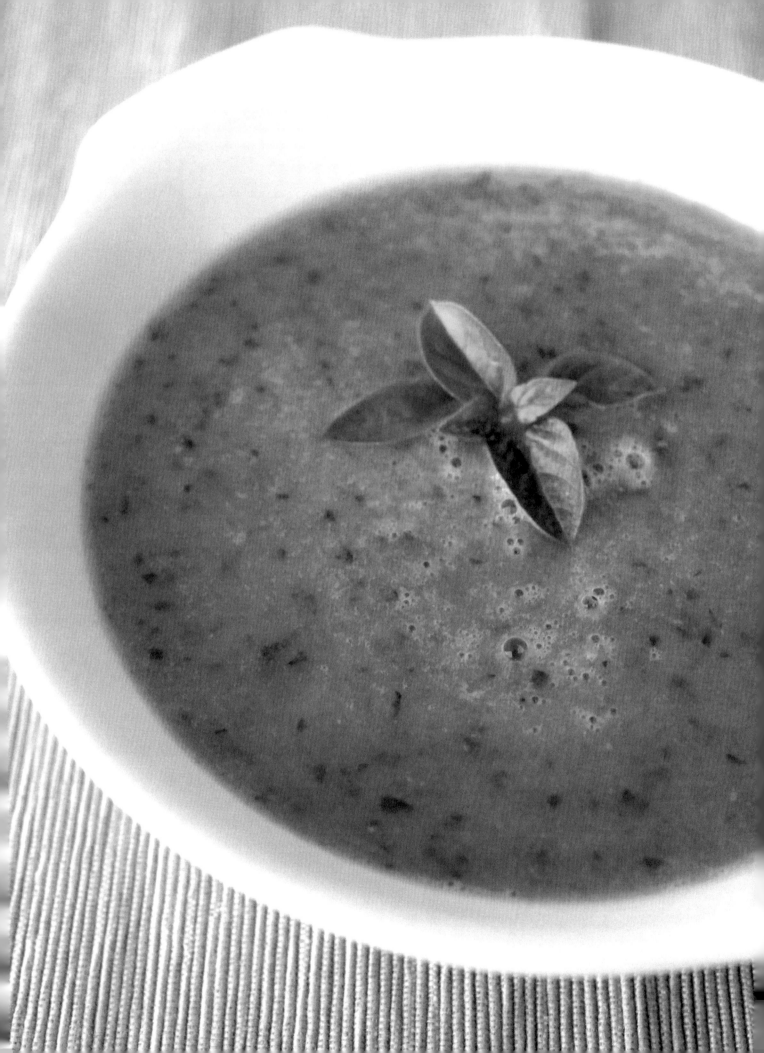

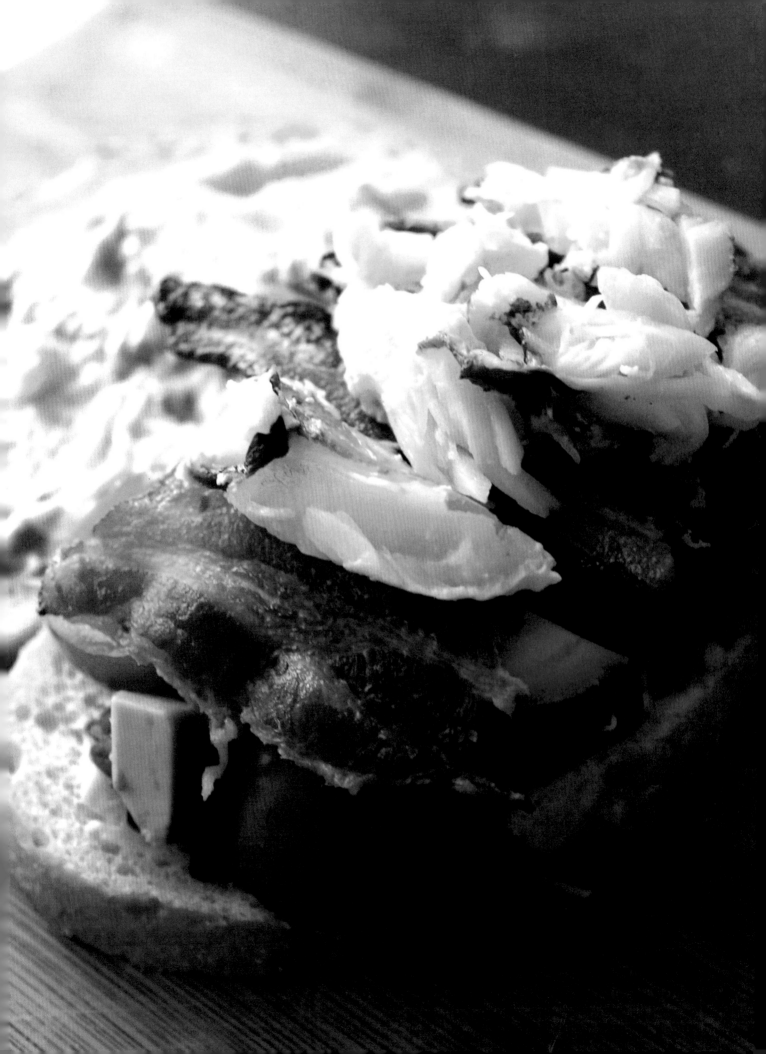

BKTAC: Bacon, kale, tomato, avocado and crab sandwich

Serves 2

6 slices thick cut bacon, cooked

1 handful baby kale or spinach

1 tomato, sliced

1 avocado, sliced

1 Dungeness crab, meat picked from shell or ¼ lb crab meat

6 roasted garlic cloves, rough chopped

3 basil leaves, cut into strips

1/4 c. mayo or vegan mayo

1/4 tsp salt

1/8 tsp pepper

Sourdough bread, sliced

In a small bowl, combine roasted garlic, basil, mayo, salt and pepper. Stir to combine, then set aside.

To assemble sandwiches, spread a layer of dressing on each slice of bread, using 4 slices total. Top 2 slices each with half the bacon, half the baby kale, half the tomato slices, half the avocado slices and half the crab. Place other bread slice on top and cut down the middle.

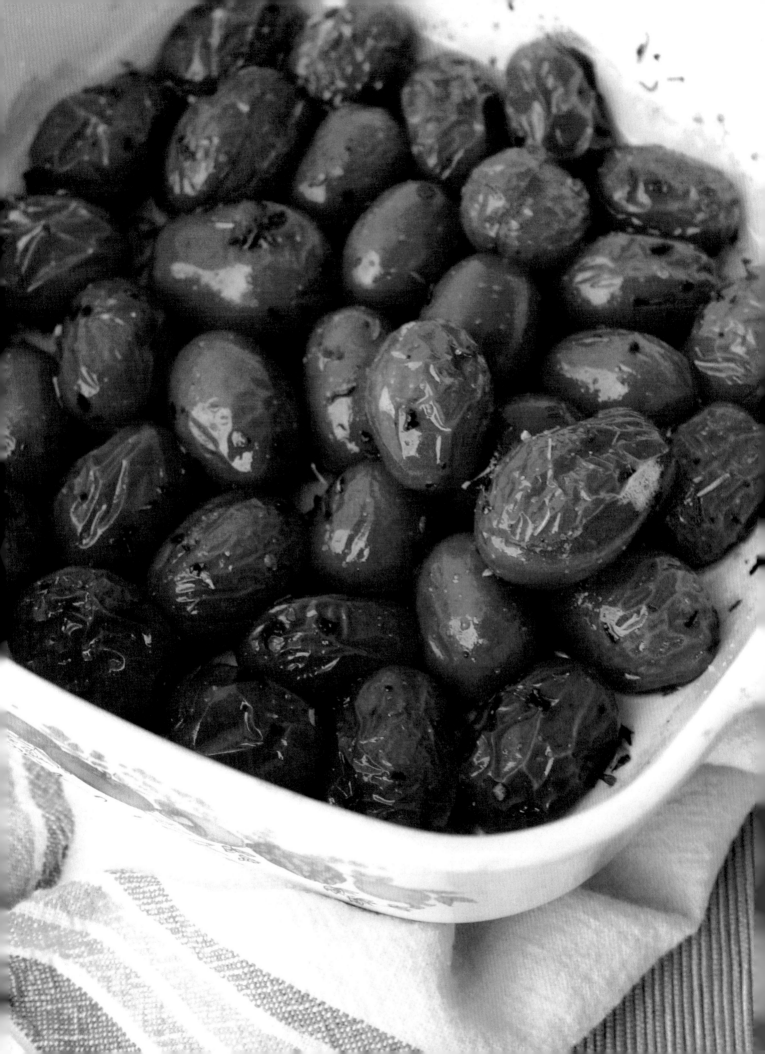

Roasted Italian Cherry Tomatoes

Serves 4

1 pint cherry tomatoes

2 tbsp olive oil

1/4 tsp Italian seasoning

1/4 tsp salt

1/8 tsp pepper

Preheat oven to 450 F. Put tomatoes into a medium ceramic baking dish, then toss with olive oil and spices. Roast in oven for 12-15 minutes until tomatoes begin to burst open.

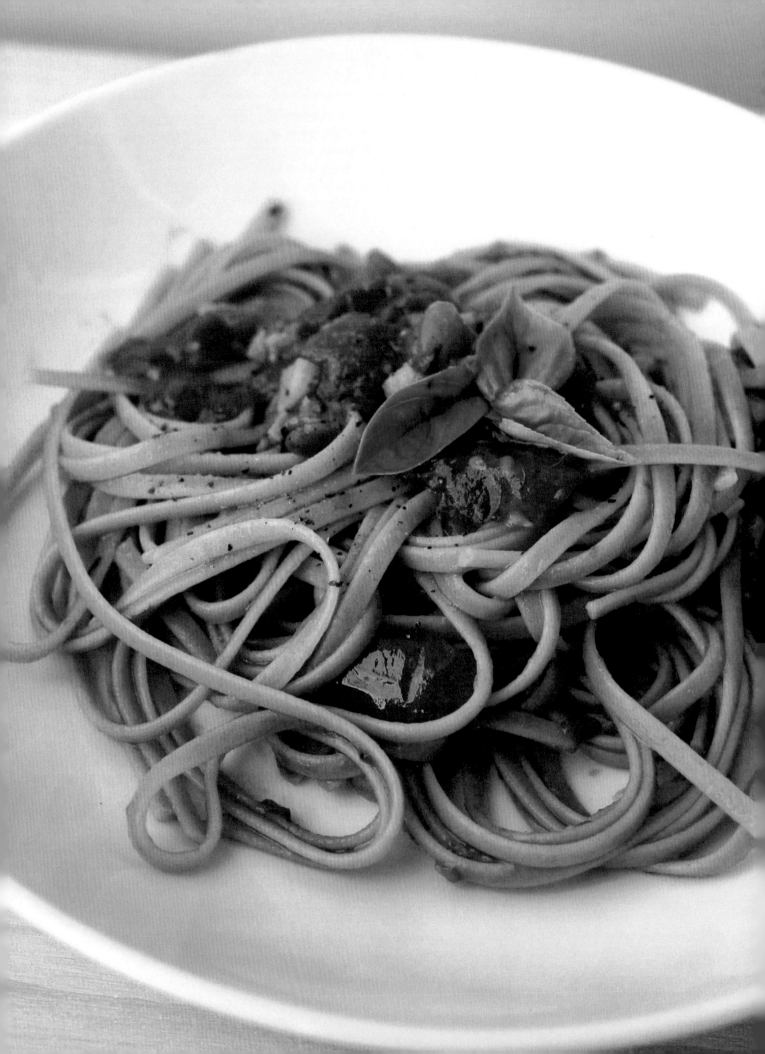

Fresh Tomato Basil Pasta

Serves 4

1 lb tomatoes, chopped

4 cloves garlic, minced

1/2 tsp each dried parsley, oregano, thyme, salt and pepper

10 fennel seeds

1/4 c. red wine

2 tsp tomato paste

Whole wheat linguine

Basil leaves

In a large stockpot, cook pasta according to package directions. Drain, reserving 1 c. of pasta water.

For sauce, heat a large sauté pan over medium heat. Add 2 tbsp olive oil, then cook garlic for 30 seconds. Add tomatoes, spices and tomato paste and cook for 5 minutes. Add wine and cook for a minute more. Add pasta to sauce along with 1/4 c. pasta water to thin sauce. Stir to combine, then serve with basil leaves sprinkled over the top.

Zucchini

I remember my mom always cooking zucchini with garlic in a sauté pan, and while it was delicious, I never knew any other way to eat it. As I learned to cook over the years, I began to explore other ways to eat zucchini.

My favorite is grilled zucchini, especially with grilled onions, which makes the grilled zucchini, tomato and onion salad with corn my favorite zucchini recipe from this book. It's a little time consuming, but it's so worth the work. And the wait!

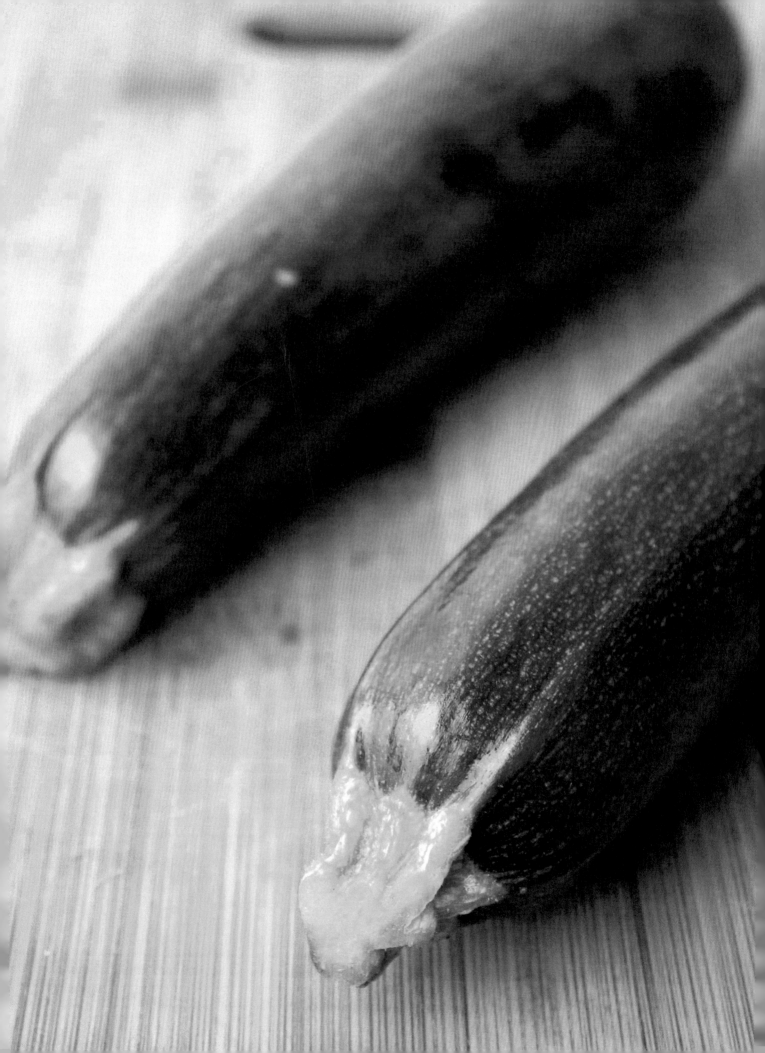

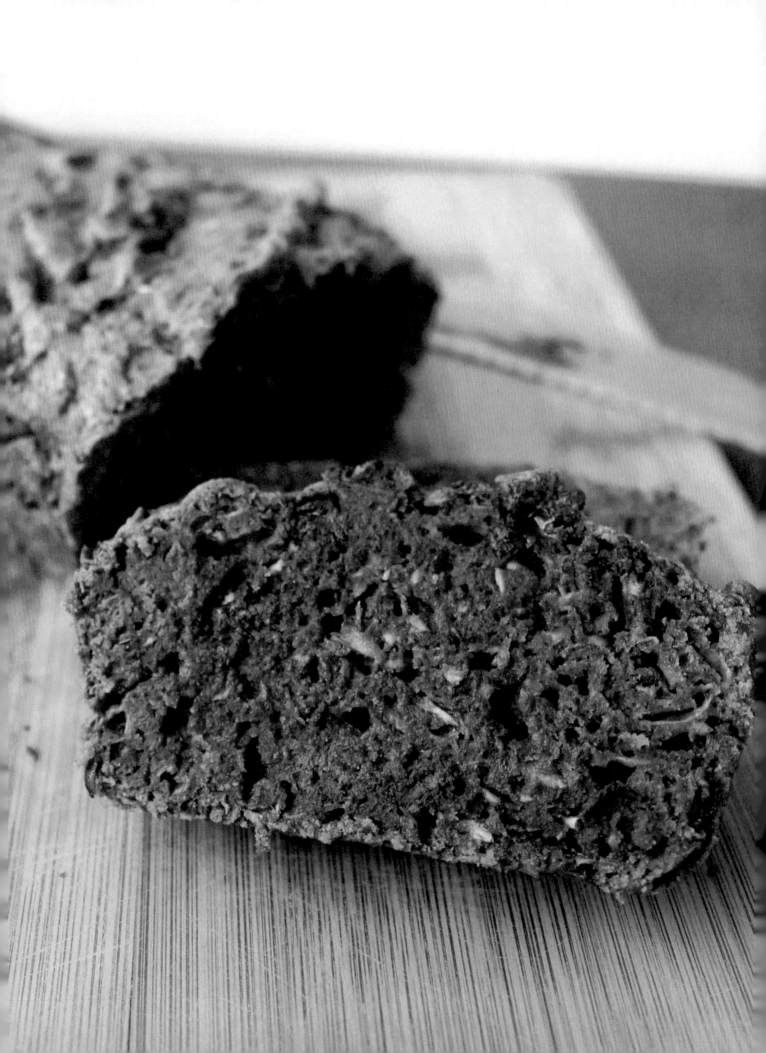

Chocolate Zucchini Bread

Makes 1 loaf

1 1/2 c. flour

3/4 tsp baking powder

1/4 tsp salt

1/4 tsp nutmeg

2 tbsp unsweetened cocoa powder, optional if you like a heavy chocolate flavor

1 tbsp ground flaxseed

3 tbsp water

2 zucchinis, shredded

3/4 c. sugar

1/2 c. oil

1/4 c. chocolate chips

Preheat oven to 350 F. Lightly grease an 8x4x2 baking pan, unless it is non-stick.

In a large bowl, combine flour, baking powder, salt, nutmeg and cocoa powder, if using. Whisk to combine, then stir in chocolate chips.

In a medium bowl, mix together shredded zucchini, sugar and oil. In a small bowl, whisk together the flaxseed and water, then pour into the bowl with the zucchini. Stir to combine, then mix with the dry ingredients with a spatula, until just moistened.

Pour batter into the baking pan and bake in the oven for 45 minutes, or until a toothpick placed in the center comes out clean. Let cool for 15 minutes before removing from pan to devour.

Zucchini and Quinoa Soup with Lemon and Thyme

Serves 4

2 zucchini, chopped

2 cloves garlic, minced

1/2 yellow onion, diced

1 c. quinoa, rinsed

4 c. chicken or vegetable stock

Zest of 1 lemon

1/2 tsp dried thyme

1/2 tsp salt

1/4 tsp pepper

In a large stock pot, heat 1 tbsp olive oil and cook garlic and onion over medium heat. Cook until onion begins to be translucent, about 3 minutes, then add zucchini. Cook another 2 minutes, then add quinoa. Stir to coat in oil, then add stock, lemon zest, and spices. Bring to a boil, then lower to a simmer and cook for 12-15 minutes, or until quinoa is just cooked. Serve hot with crusty bread.

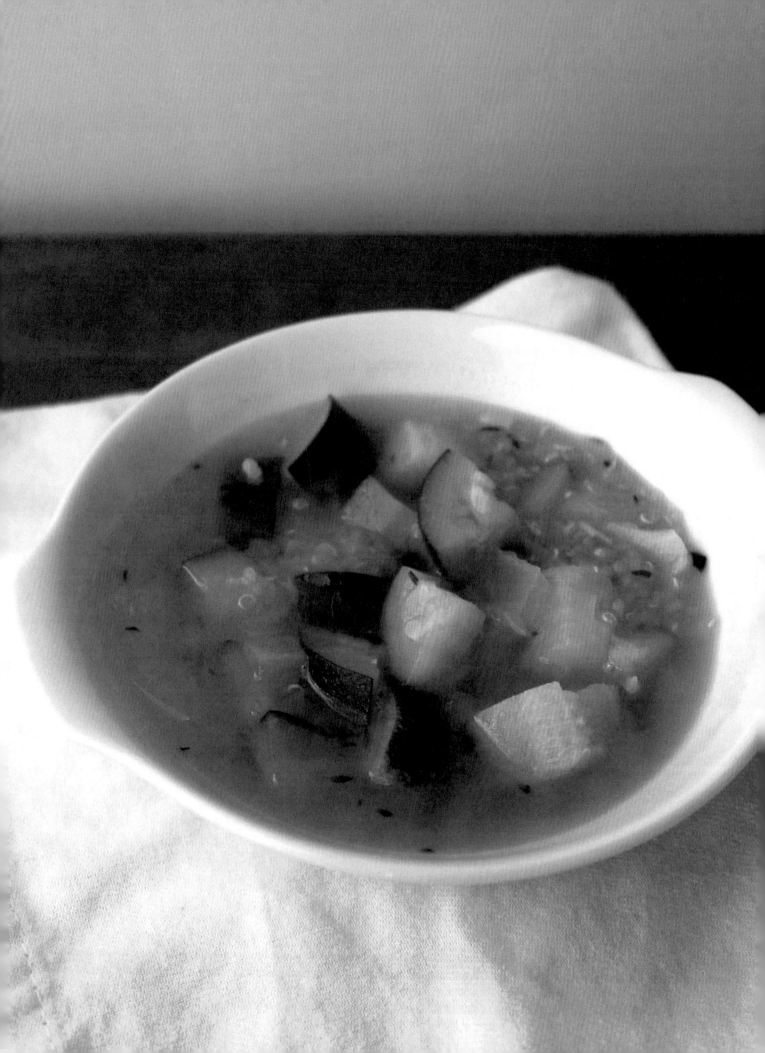

Grilled Corn, Tomato, Zucchini and Sweet Onion Salad

Serves 4

1 yellow onion, thinly sliced

2 zucchini, sliced lengthwise into long ribbons, or just cut in half lengthwise

2 tomatoes, cut in half

1 c. frozen corn, thawed, or 1 ear corn

2 cloves garlic, minced

Olive oil

1/2 tsp salt

1/4 tsp pepper

Heat a grill or grill pan to medium high heat. If using an ear of corn, pull the husks and silk off, then brush with olive oil. Place ear directly on the grill and cook, turning every few minutes to nicely brown the corn. When all the kernels are cooked, let cool until you can cut off the kernels. Add to the bowl with the zucchini.

Toss zucchini in olive oil, then grill slices, doing them in several batches. Each piece of zucchini takes about 2 minutes to cook per side. Flip each zucchini to get grill marks on both sides. Add zucchini to a large bowl.

Once zucchini are grilled, grill tomato halves with the cut side down. Cook for 3 minutes, then flip and cook for 3 more. Set aside to cool, then cut into wedges and add to bowl with the zucchini.

In a sauté pan, heat 1 tbsp olive oil over medium heat and grill onions for 5-7 minutes or until they are nicely browned. Set aside in the bowl with the zucchini. Add garlic and corn kernels, if using, and sauté until garlic and corn kernels are browned, about 1-2 minutes. Pour into bowl the rest of the veggies and toss to combine. Serve either hot or chilled.

*For a less labor intensive version, just cut each zucchini in half lengthwise then grill the halves until cooked through, about 5-7 minutes total. Once cool, slice into half-moons.

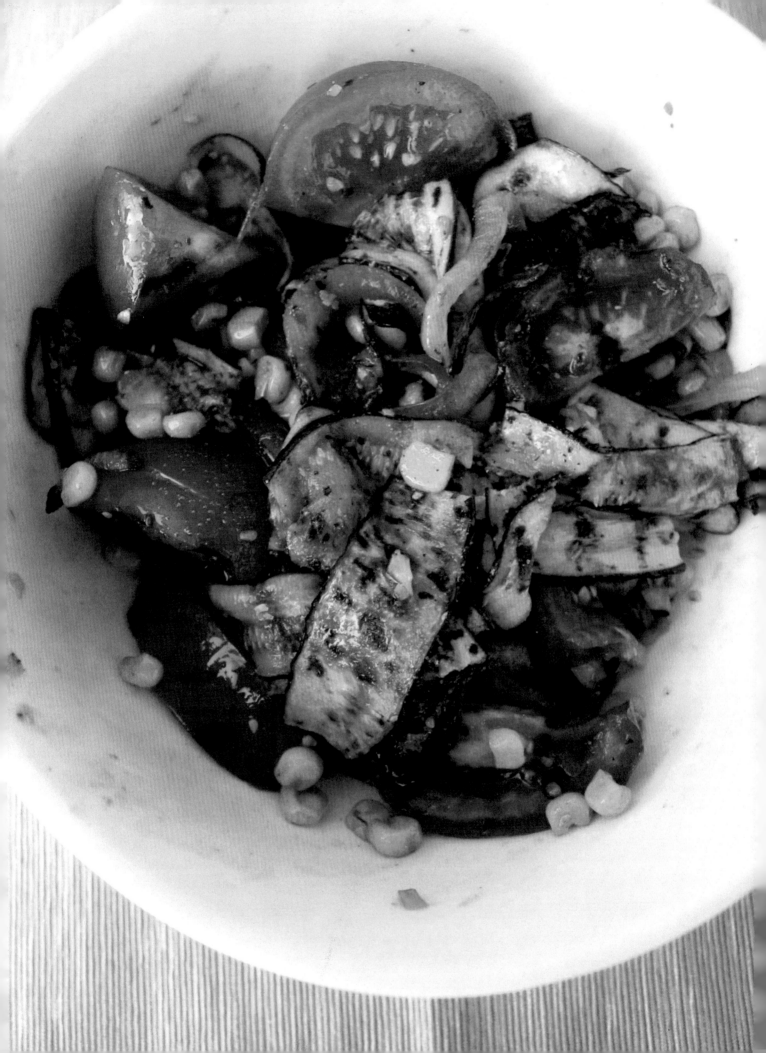

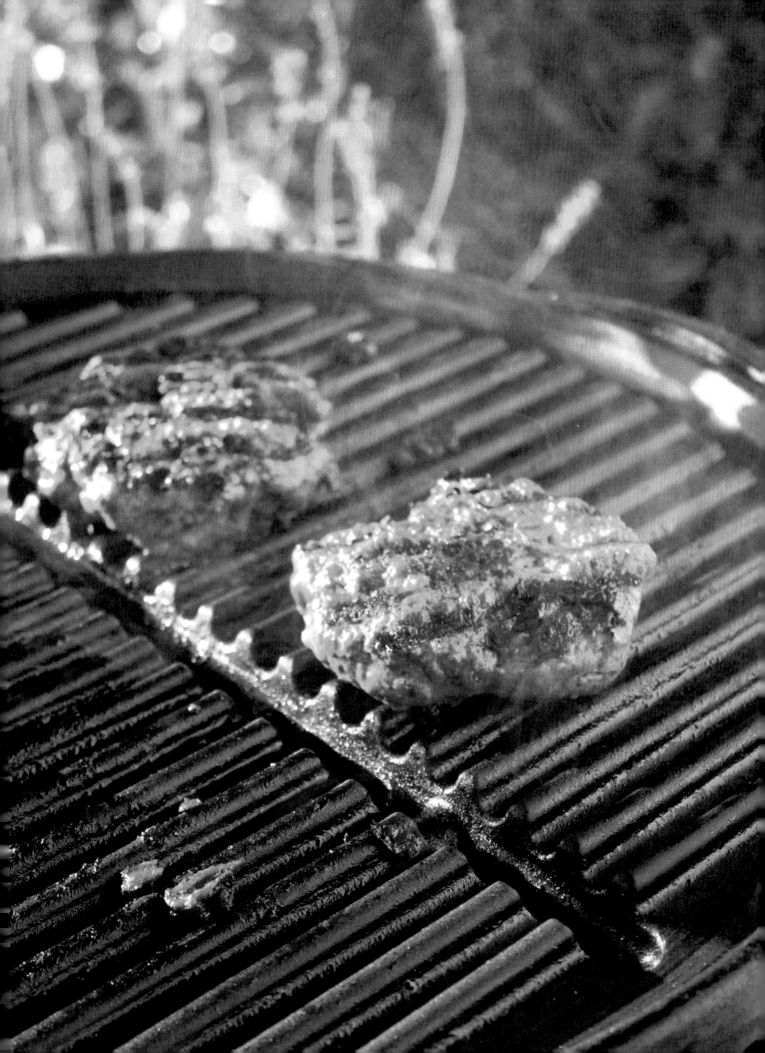

Baked Zucchinis and Tomatoes with Panko Crust

Serves 4

2 zucchinis, cubed

4 medium tomatoes, each cut into 6 wedges

2 tbsp olive oil

1 clove garlic, minced

1/2 tsp salt

1/4 tsp pepper

1/4 c. panko or breadcrumbs

Preheat oven to 400 F. In a bowl, combine zucchini, tomatoes, garlic, spices and oil and toss to coat. Pour into a large baking dish and sprinkle the top with the panko. Bake for 20-25 minutes, or until zucchini is cooked and the panko is golden brown.

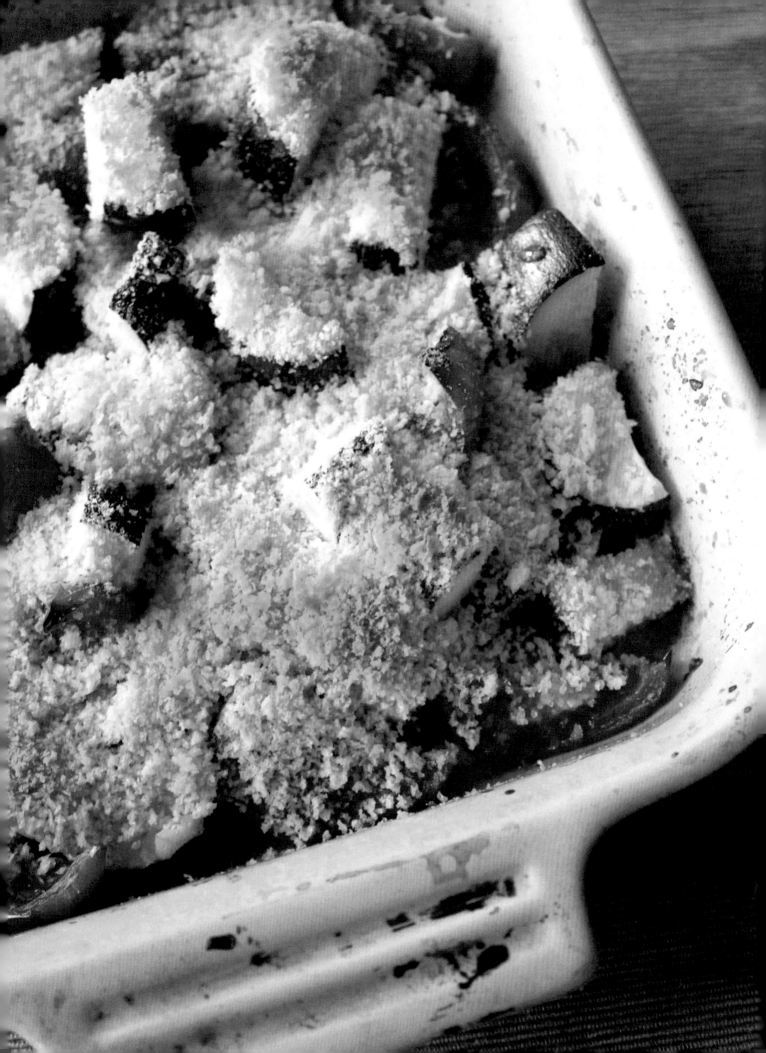

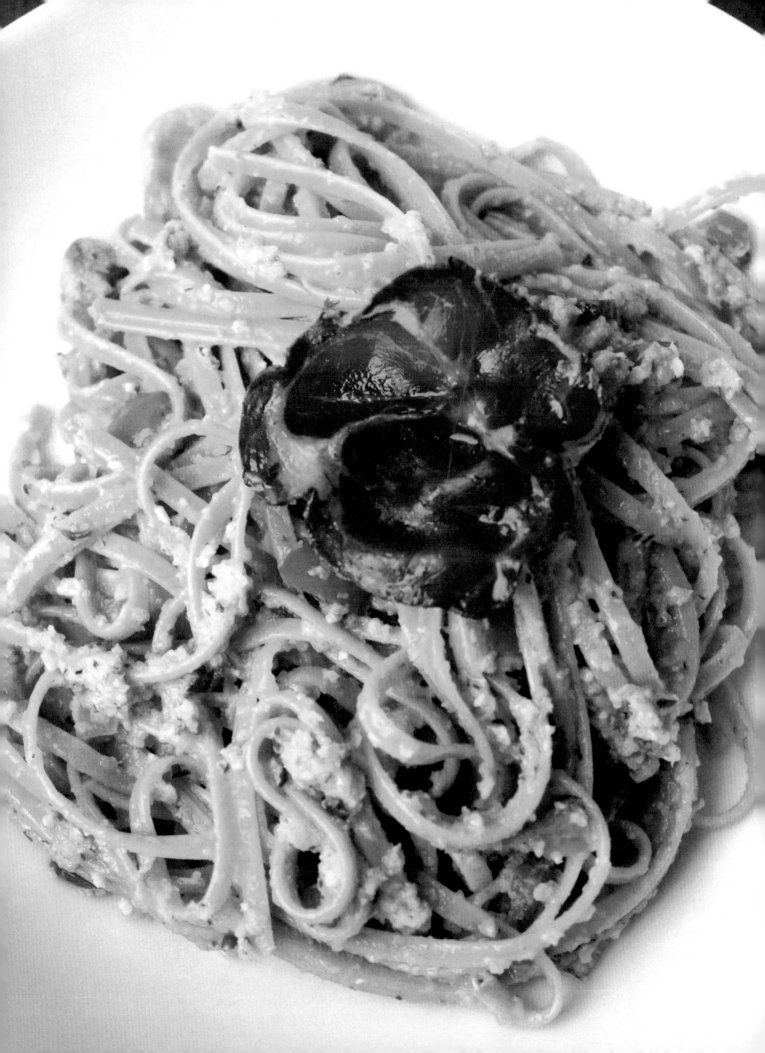

Zucchini Pesto Pasta with Crispy Coppa

Serves 4

2 zucchinis, trimmed and cut in quarters

2 cloves garlic

10 basil leaves

1/2 tsp salt

1/4 tsp pepper

1/4 c. pine nuts

1/4 c. olive oil

1 red bell pepper, small diced

Linguine

8 slices coppa or prosciutto

Preheat oven to 350 F. Lay a piece of parchment paper on a baking sheet, then place coppa or prosciutto slices on it. Bake for 5-6 minutes until nice and crispy. Remove from oven and let cool.

Bring a large pot of water to a boil. Cook linguine according to package directions. Drain and set aside.

Grate zucchini and garlic cloves in a food processor. Heat large sauté pan over medium heat, then add 1 tbsp oil. Pour zucchini and garlic mixture into the pan and cook for 3-4 minutes until zucchini is cooked through. Return to food processor, along with basil, pine nuts, salt, pepper and olive oil. Process until emulsified.

In the same pan you cooked the zucchini in, cook the bell pepper cubes over medium high heat for 1-2 minutes until crisp tender. Add pesto and pasta to pan and toss to combine. Divide onto four plates and top each with 1-2 pieces of crispy coppa.

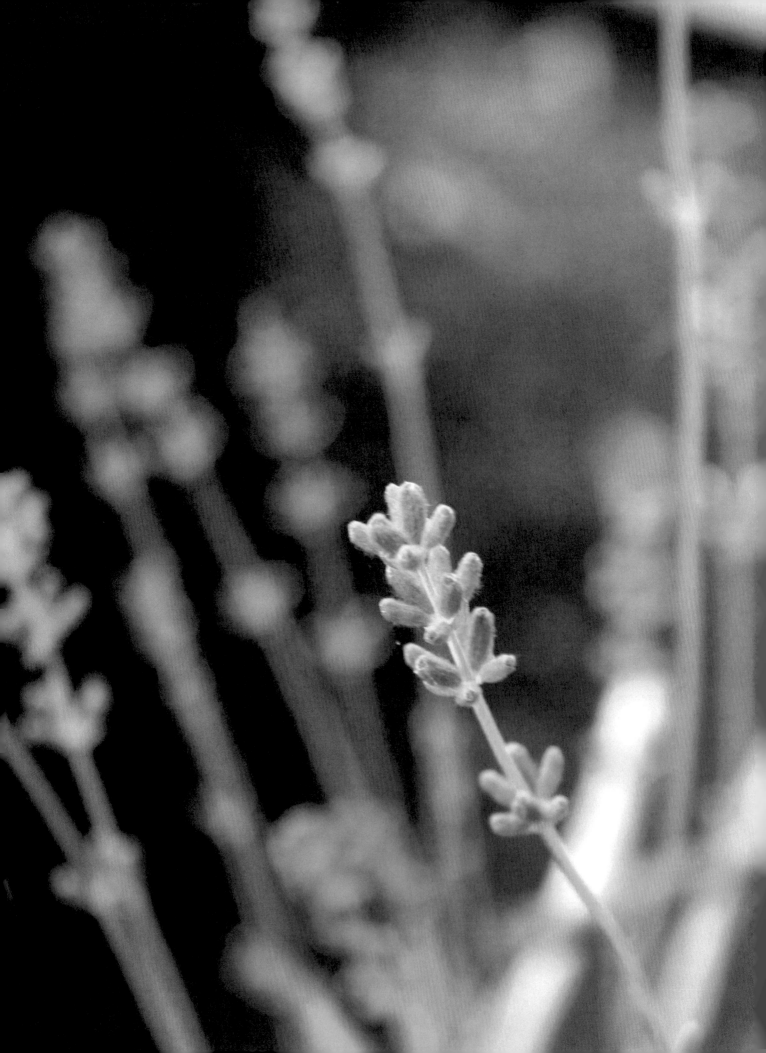

Summer Fruits

Stone fruits and berries are the highlight of summer fruits. Cherries, apricots, peaches and nectarines arc all delicious eaten straight from the tree and need hardly any embellishment. Berries are the same way. I love collecting blackberries from bushes that grow wild here and gobbling them up. They make such good desserts and snacks all by themselves.

Of course, I had to add a little bit more to them because otherwise it wouldn't be considered cooking! Most of the recipes in here are so simple and quick that you can enjoy them every night of the week. From cakes to granitas to simple fruit salads, there is a fruit recipe in this book perfect for anyone.

Apricots

I would have to say that apricots are my favorite summer fruit. I search for them every spring at my grocery store and simply cannot wait to spot those little golden globes of sweetness. In fact, I buy so many sometimes they run out. When I can't find fresh ones, I'll always go for some dried apricots to get my sweet fix. They are perfect as an awesome trail mix addition.

My favorite way to eat apricots is definitely to stew them then stir them into oatmeal or serve them over granola. On a cool morning, I'll whip up a batch of stewed apricots so I can make my mornings a little easier and a little brighter with their cheery color.

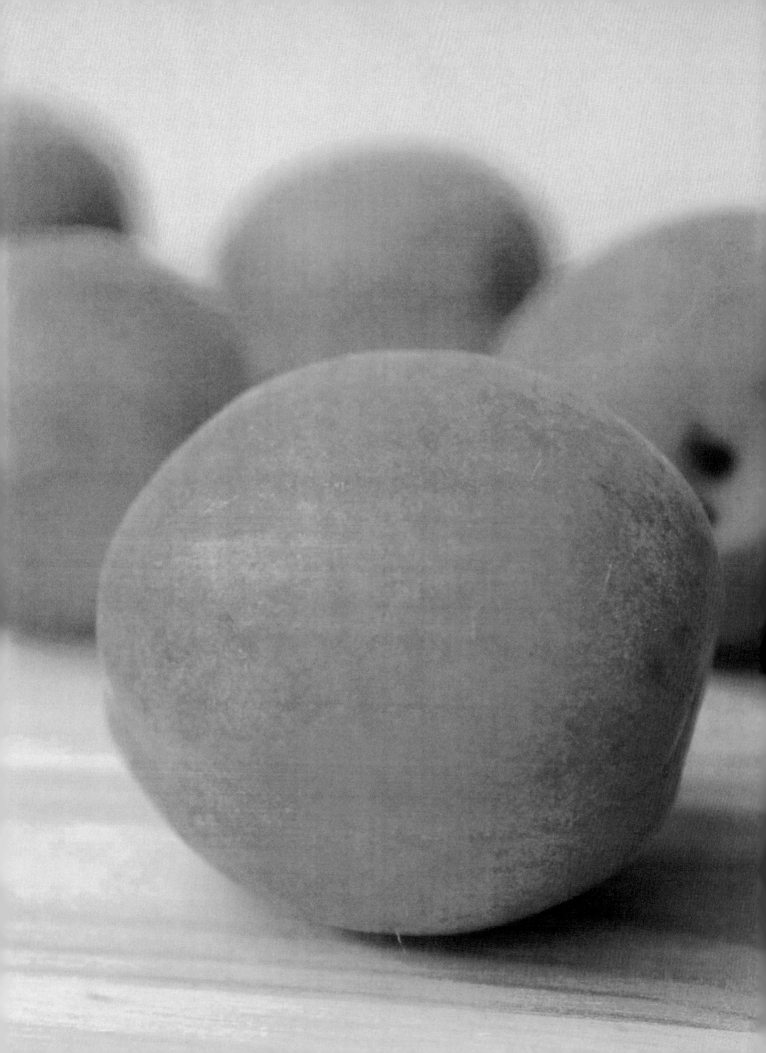

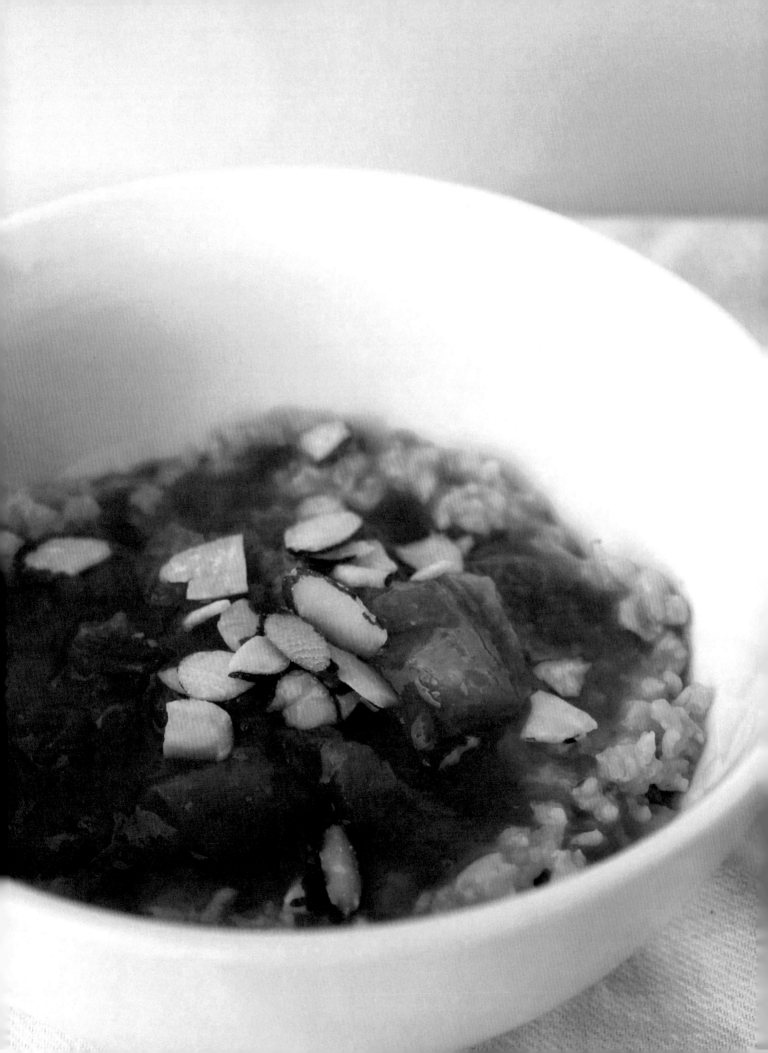

Spiced Apricots over Oatmeal

Makes 2 servings, plus extra apricots

For spiced apricots:

5 apricots, pitted and diccd

1 clove

1 cardamom seed

1/2 cinnamon stick

1/4 c. sugar

1/2 c. apricot nectar

2/3 c. rolled oats (not instant)

1 tbsp brown sugar

1/8 tsp salt

Water

To make spiced apricots, combine all ingredients in a medium saucepan, bring to a boil, then reduce to a simmer. Cook for 5 minutes, or until apricots begin to break down. Set aside to cool.

For oatmeal, in a medium saucepan, combine all ingredients, including enough water to cover the oats by about 1/2". Turn burner onto medium high, set timer for 5 minutes and let cook. When timer goes off, remove from heat and let stand another 5 minutes to let liquid absorb.

Spoon oatmeal into bowls, then top with a healthy spoonful of the spiced apricots.

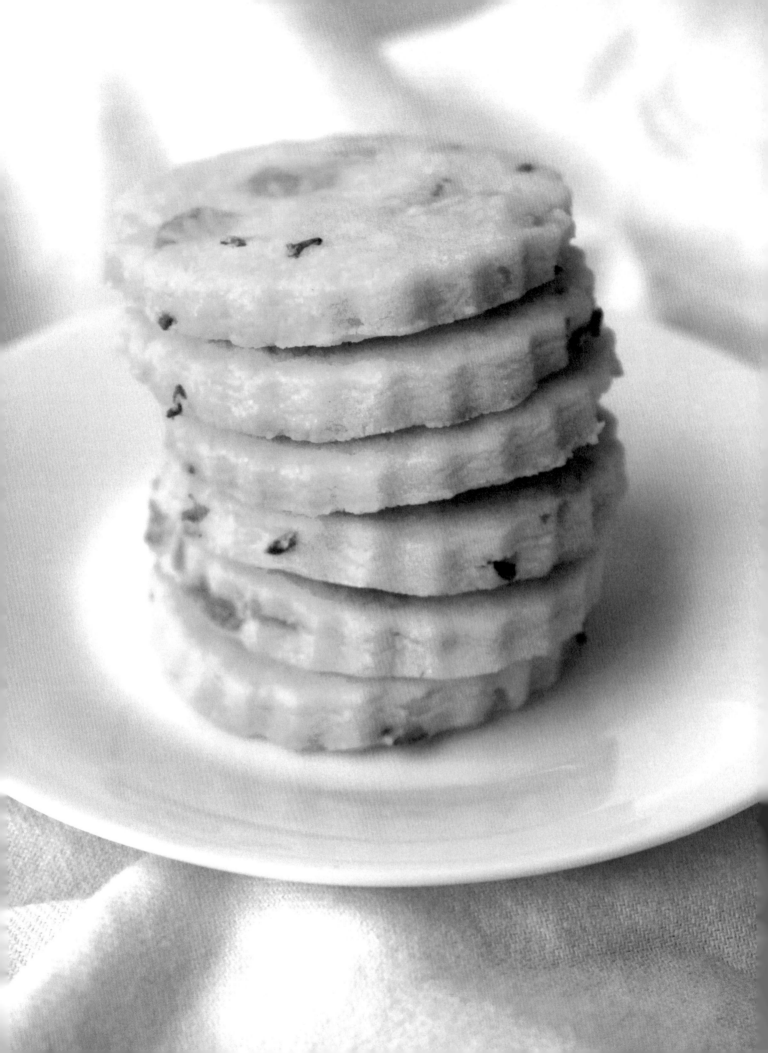

Apricot Sugar Cookies with Lavender

Makes 3 dozen cookies

10 dried apricots, finely diced

2 c. AP flour

1/4 tsp salt

1 tbsp dried lavender

3/4 c. butter or vegan butter, softened

3/4 c. sugar

1 1/2 tsp Ener-G egg replacer plus 2 tbsp warm water or 1 egg

1 tsp vanilla extract

In a medium bowl, combine flour, salt and lavender. Whisk together egg replacer and water, then set aside. Using a stand mixer, cream butter and sugar on high speed until the butter turns a sunny yellow and becomes a little fluffy, about 2 minutes. Add egg replacer or egg and vanilla extract and beat for 30 seconds on medium, until just combined, scraping sides down if necessary.

Add flour mixture and apricots, and beat on low speed until just combined. Scrape down sides, then cover with plastic wrap. Chill in the refrigerator for at least 1 hour.

Heat oven to 350F. Roll dough out on a floured surface to 1/4" thick. Cut into desired shapes then place on ungreased baking sheet. Bake for 13 minutes, or until barely golden on the edges. Cool for a few minutes on the sheet, then remove to a cooling rack to cool until eaten.

Apricot Bread

Makes 1 loaf

1 3/4 c. AP flour

1/3 c. sugar

2 tsp baking powder

1/4 tsp salt

1 1/2 tsp Ener-G Egg Replacer Powder plus 2 tbsp warm water or 1 egg, slightly beaten

3/4 c. apricot nectar

1/4 c. oil

4 apricots, pitted and diced

Preheat oven to 400 F. Grease a 8x4x2 baking pan, unless nonstick.

In a large bowl, combine flour, sugar, baking powder and salt. Whisk to combine. In a small bowl, combine egg replacer powder with the warm water and whisk to mix. Set aside.

In a medium bowl, combine apricot nectar, oil and apricots. Stir to mix, then stir in the egg replacer mixture or 1 egg. Pour into the dry ingredients, and stir until moistened. Pour batter into the baking pan and bake in the oven for 45-50 minutes, or until a toothpick placed in the center comes out clean. Let cool for 15 minutes in the pan before removing and slicing.

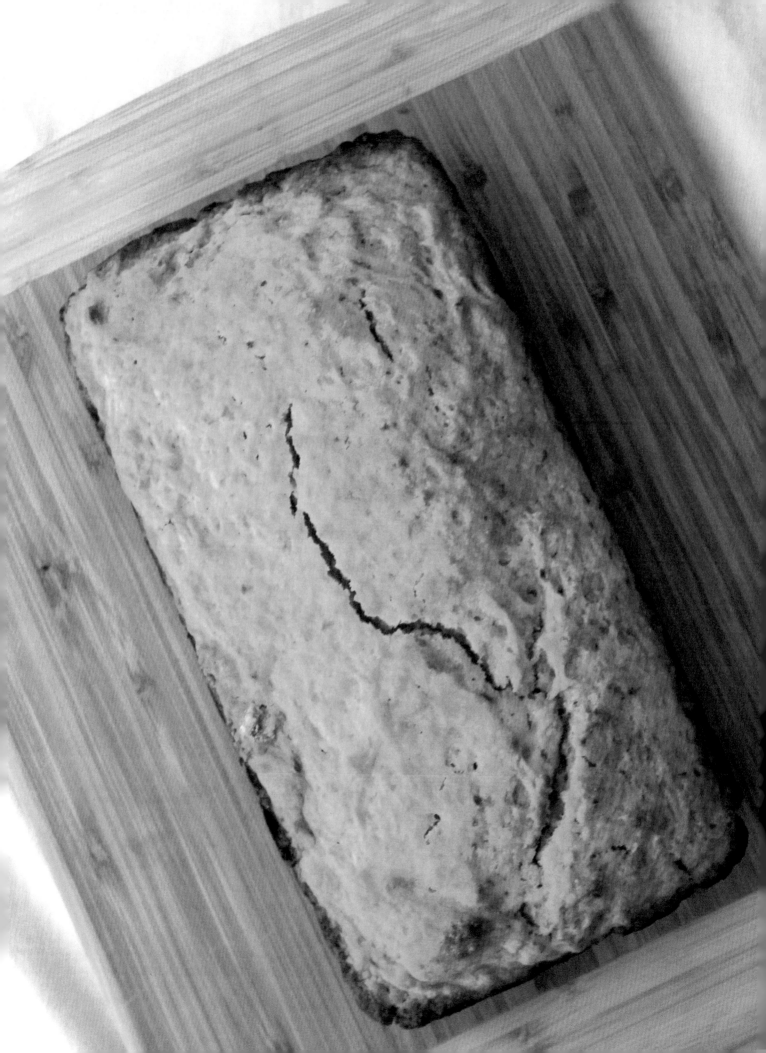

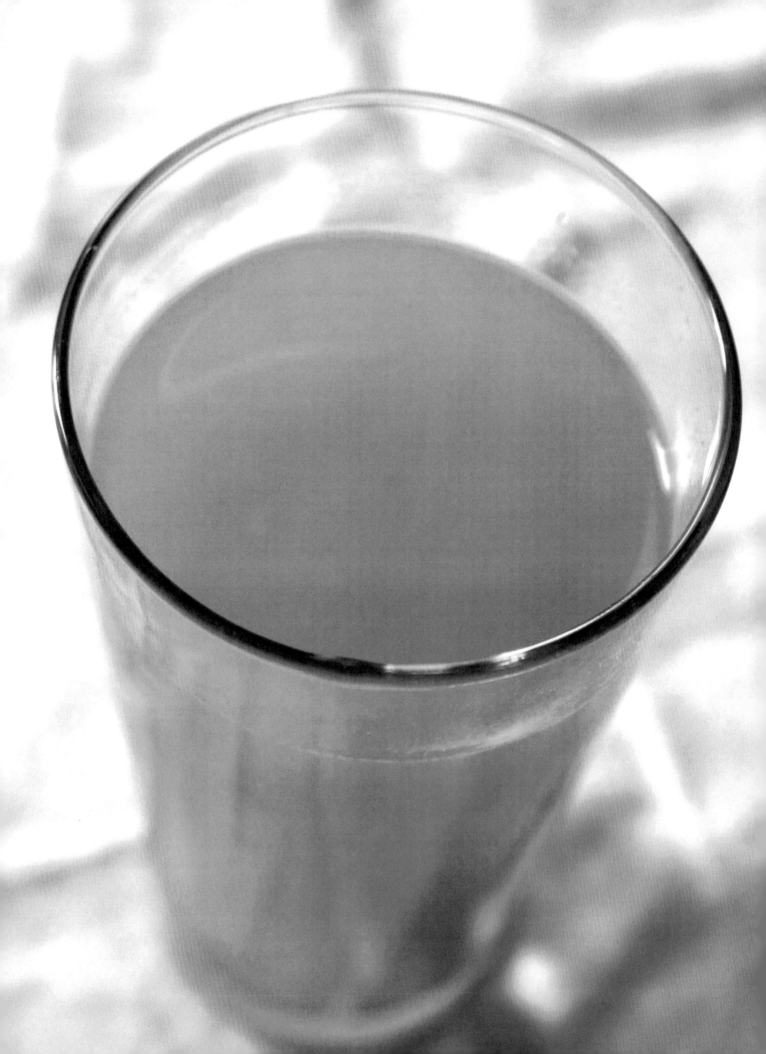

Apricot Vanilla Soda

Makes 2 drinks

1 c. apricot nectar
2 tbsp vanilla syrup
ice
sparkling water

Vanilla syrup:
1/2 c. water
1/2 c. sugar
1 vanilla bean pod, split open (or 1 tsp vanilla extract)

To make vanilla syrup, combine all ingredients in a saucepan. Bring to a boil, and stir until sugar is dissolved then remove from heat to cool. Store in a glass jar. Makes about 1 c. vanilla syrup.

For soda, in each glass, stir together 1/2 c. apricot nectar and 1 tbsp vanilla syrup. Add ice and fill glass with sparkling water. Add more syrup for a sweeter taste, if desired.

Apricot Blueberry Wild Rice Pilaf

Serves 4

1 box wild rice pilaf (I like the Near East brand)

1 tsp ground sage

Salt and pepper

½ c. blueberries

2 apricots, diced

Cook rice according to package directions, substituting in the sage and salt and pepper for the seasoning mix. After the rice is cooked, stir in the blueberries and apricots and serve.

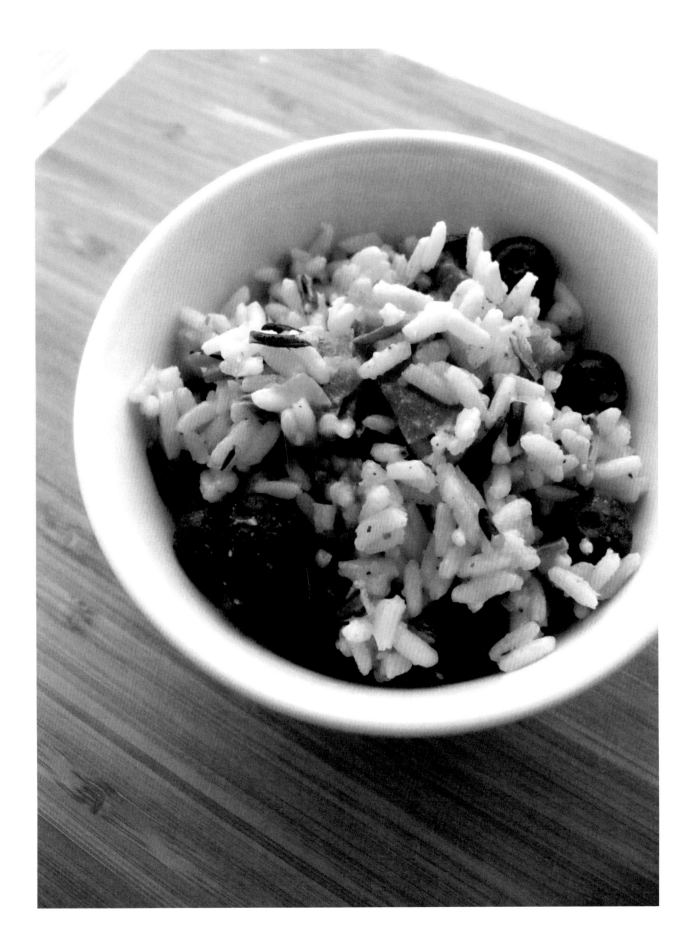

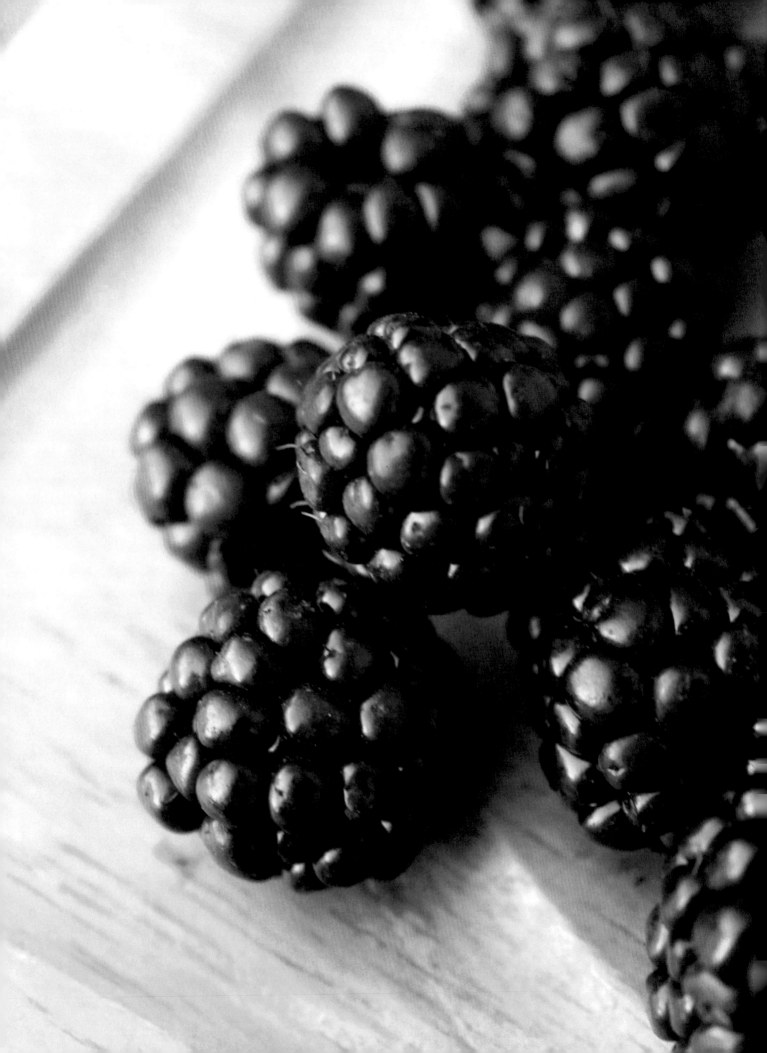

Dark Berries

Blueberries and blackberries. Aren't they just so yummy? I have very distinct memories of picking both. My grandparents grew blueberries in their backyard and whenever us grandkids were getting rowdy, my grandma would hand us a bucket and tell us to pick until the buckets were full. She counted on us eating almost as many as we picked, but then we almost always got blueberry pancakes the next morning, which were a treat.

Blackberries, on the other hand, grow wild here so much that it's almost impossible to get rid of them. So we just pick the berries and do our best to keep them at bay. I remember going along this road around the corner from where I grew up to pick them, always being careful not to get poked by the thorns.

My favorite dark berry recipe is the blackberry lemon cake. It's a dense sponge cake that has blackberries popping out of it. This cake is perfect for any dessert, and is also great for breakfast.

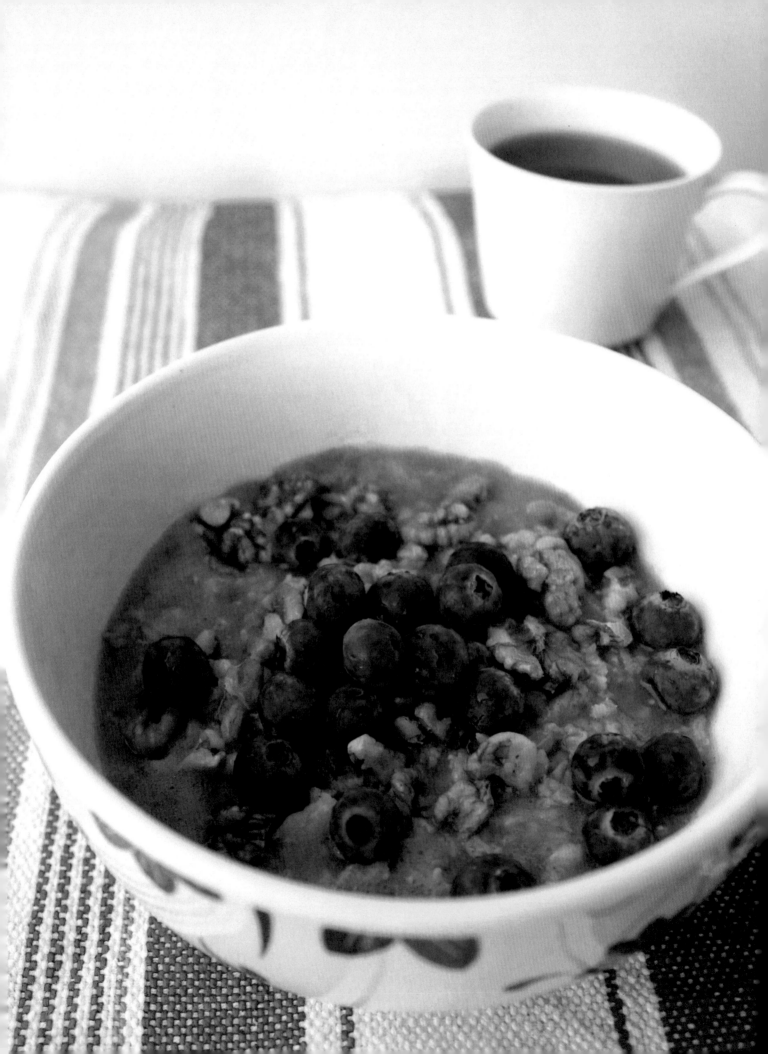

Blueberry and Walnut Oatmeal

Serves 1

1/3 c. regular rolled oats (not instant)

1 tbsp brown sugar

1 tsp cinnamon

1/8 tsp salt

Water, to cover

Blueberries

Walnuts

Almond milk, optional

In a medium saucepan, combine oats, sugar, cinnamon and salt. Add enough water to cover by ½". Start timer for 5 minutes and bring to a boil. Cook until timer goes off. Remove from heat and let stand for 1 minute to cool. Pour into a bowl, then top with a handful each of blueberries and walnuts. Add a splash of almond milk to thin out and cool down, if too thick.

Blackberry Yogurt Fool with Peaches

Serves 4

2 containers plain coconut yogurt

½ pint blackberries, rinsed and drained

2 peaches, peeled, pitted and diced

Granola or crumbled cookies, if desired

Pour blackberries into a large bowl, then mash slightly with a potato masher or a spoon, just enough to break them into smaller pieces but not puree. Add coconut yogurt and gently fold blackberries into yogurt using a spatula.

Chill blackberry yogurt mixture for at least an hour. To serve, separate into 4 bowls and top each with some diced peaches and some granola or crumbled cookies.

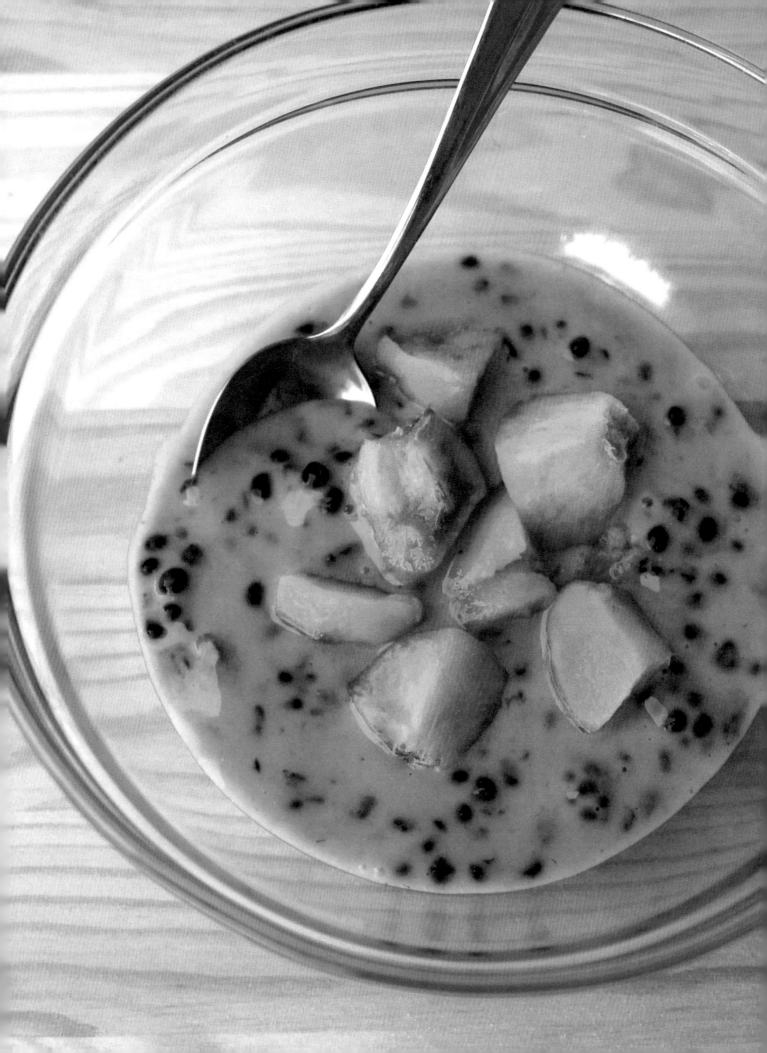

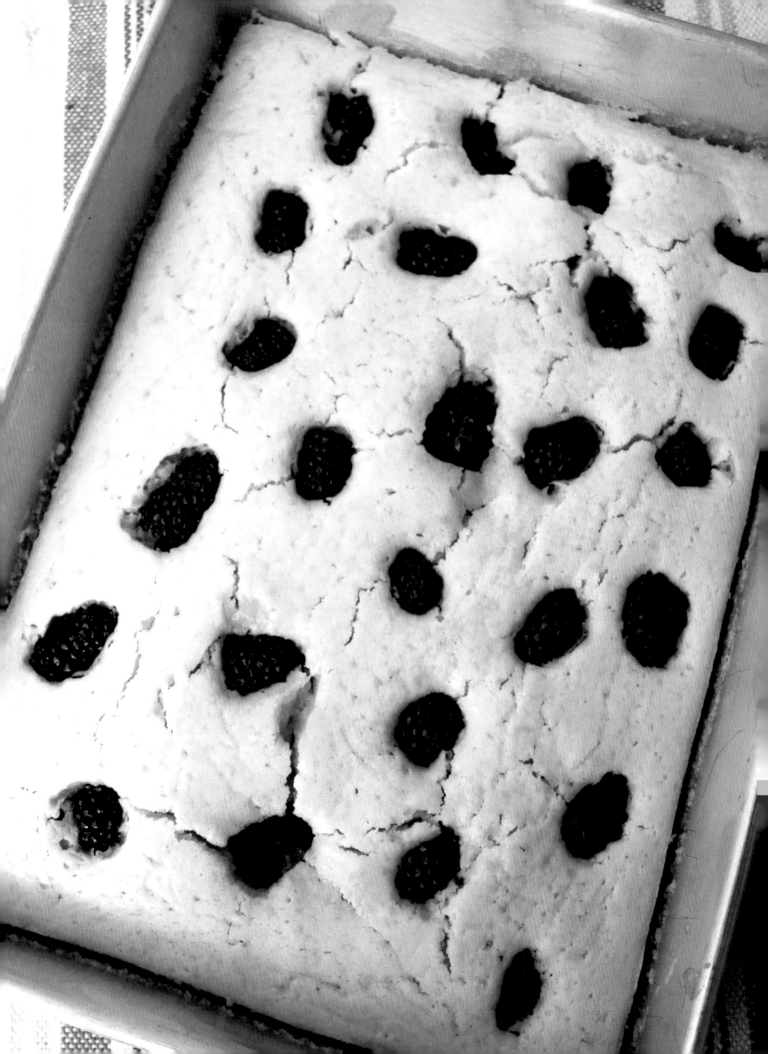

Blackberry Lemon Cake

Makes 1 sheet cake

¾ c. Earth Balance or butter, left at room temp for 15 min

4 ½ tsp Ener-G egg replacer or 3 eggs

2 ½ c. cake flour or 2 ¼ c. AP flour plus ¼ c. cornstarch, sifted

2 ½ tsp baking powder

½ tsp salt

1 ¾ c. sugar

1 tsp vanilla

1 ¼ c. soy or almond milk plus 1 tbsp white vinegar

Zest of 1 lemon

½ pint blackberries, rinsed and dried

Heat oven to 375 F. Grease bottom of a 13x9x2 inch pan. Set aside. Mix together egg replacer with ¼ c. plus 2 tbsp warm water and set aside. Mix together milk, vinegar, lemon zest and vanilla in a bowl, then set aside. Mix flour, baking powder and salt together.

In a bowl of a stand mixer, beat butter on high for 30 seconds. Add sugar ½ c. at a time and beat at medium speed until mixture becomes crumbly and sugar is mixed in. Beat on medium speed for 2 more minutes, then add egg mixture, half at a time. Add ½ c. at a time of flour mixture and milk mixture at low speed, alternating, waiting for flour to be incorporated before adding more. Batter should have a nice yellow color and be only slightly runny.

Pour batter into greased pan, spreading to even it out. Scatter blackberries over the top, then bake for 25-30 minutes, until wooden toothpick comes clean. Cool for at least 45 minutes, then serve.

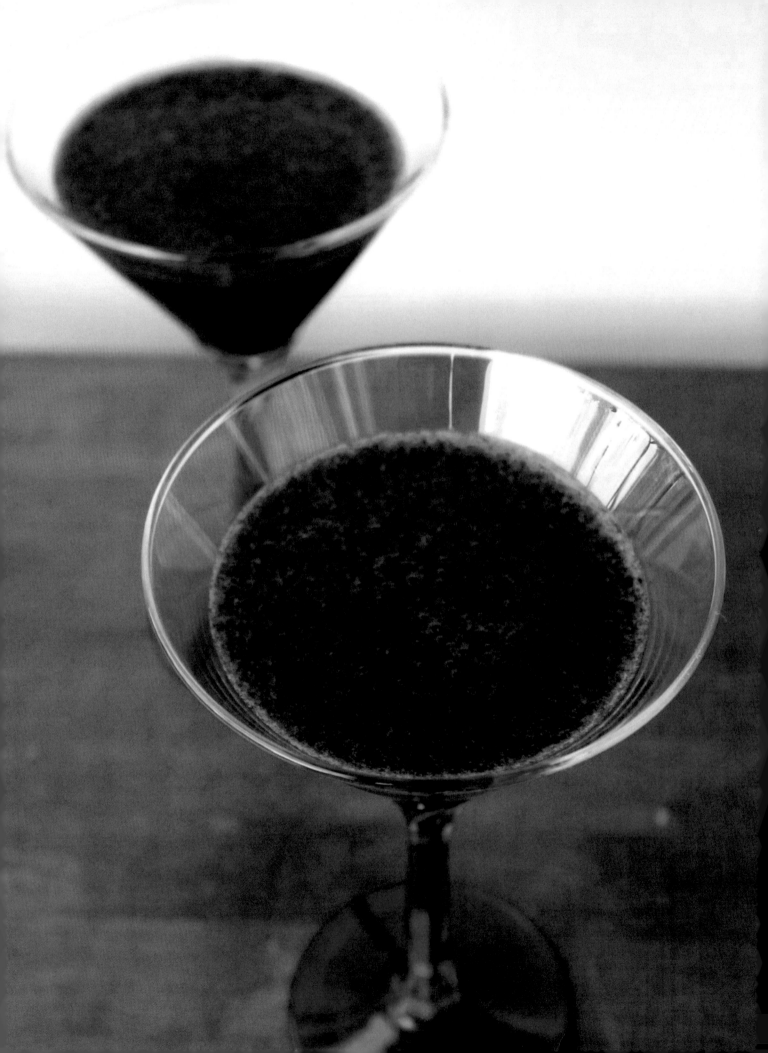

Black and Blue Martini

Makes 2 drinks

1/2 pint blackberries

1/2 pint blueberries

2 tbsp simple syrup

2 oz vodka

Ice

In a blender, combine berries and puree. Strain through a mesh strainer, reserving juice.

To make drinks, combine half of the juice, simple syrup, vodka and 3 cubes of ice in a cocktail shaker. Shake to combine and chill, then strain into 2 martini glasses.

Blueberry Sauce over Steak

Serves 4

Your favorite cut of steak

1/2 pint blueberries, rinsed

1/2 small onion, thinly sliced

1/4 c. beef broth

1/4 tsp sage

1/4 tsp salt

1/8 tsp pepper

Heat a large sauté pan over medium high heat. Sprinkle with salt and pepper, and sear steak, turning once. After steaks are cooked to your liking, set aside and keep warm.

Add onion to the pan and sauté until it begins to turn golden, about 2-3 minutes. Add berries and cook until they begin to pop and release their juices, about 3 minutes. Gently push on the berries to get them to pop if need be, but be careful because they may squirt directly at you!

Add broth to the pan and let simmer for another 2-3 minutes until slightly reduced. Add sage, salt and pepper, then carefully pour into a blender. Blend until smooth, then pour over the steaks. Serve with a green salad and potatoes.

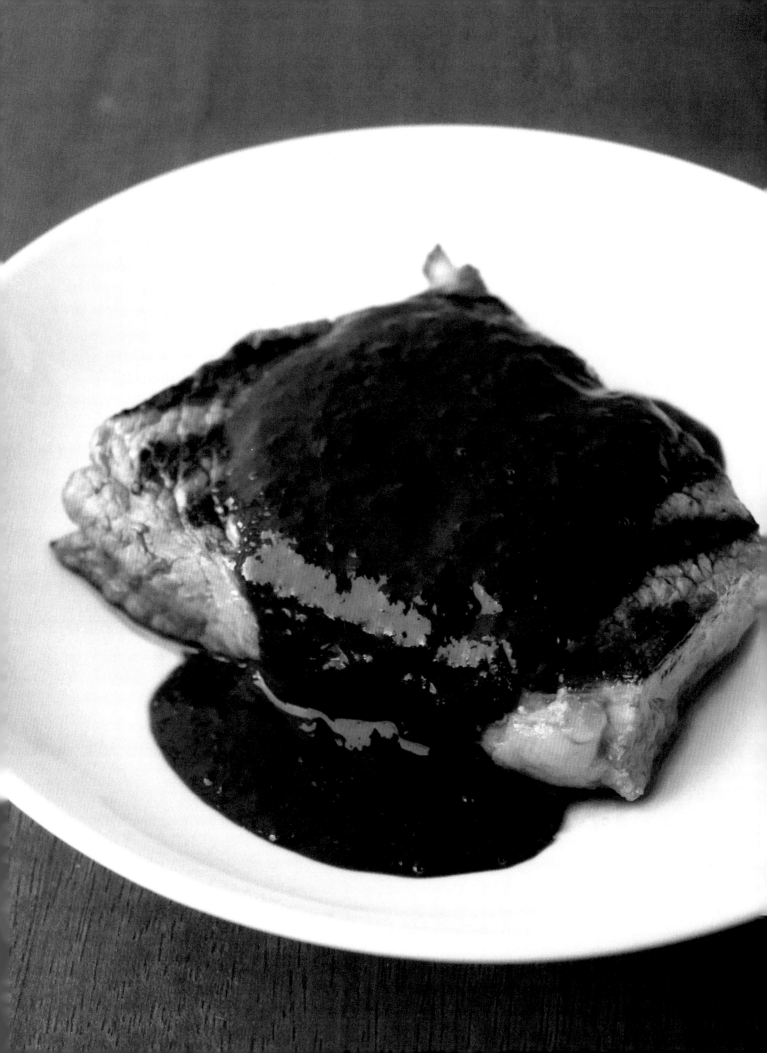

Cherries

Oh cherries. I would just be perfectly content sitting outside under a cherry tree, eating as many as I could pick from its lower branches. I loved picking cherries when I was little, although I do think the squirrels got more of them than I ever did! Still, they were delicious.

My favorite way to eat cherries when I was little was my grandma's bublanina, which translates roughly as "bubble cake." This was because the cherries were placed on top of the cake batter before baking and would look like bubbles in the cake.

Now I love my cherries in a crisp, with that delicious cinnamon oat topping that I just can't get enough of. The recipe in this book is meant for 2, but who am I kidding? It's too good to share with anyone else!

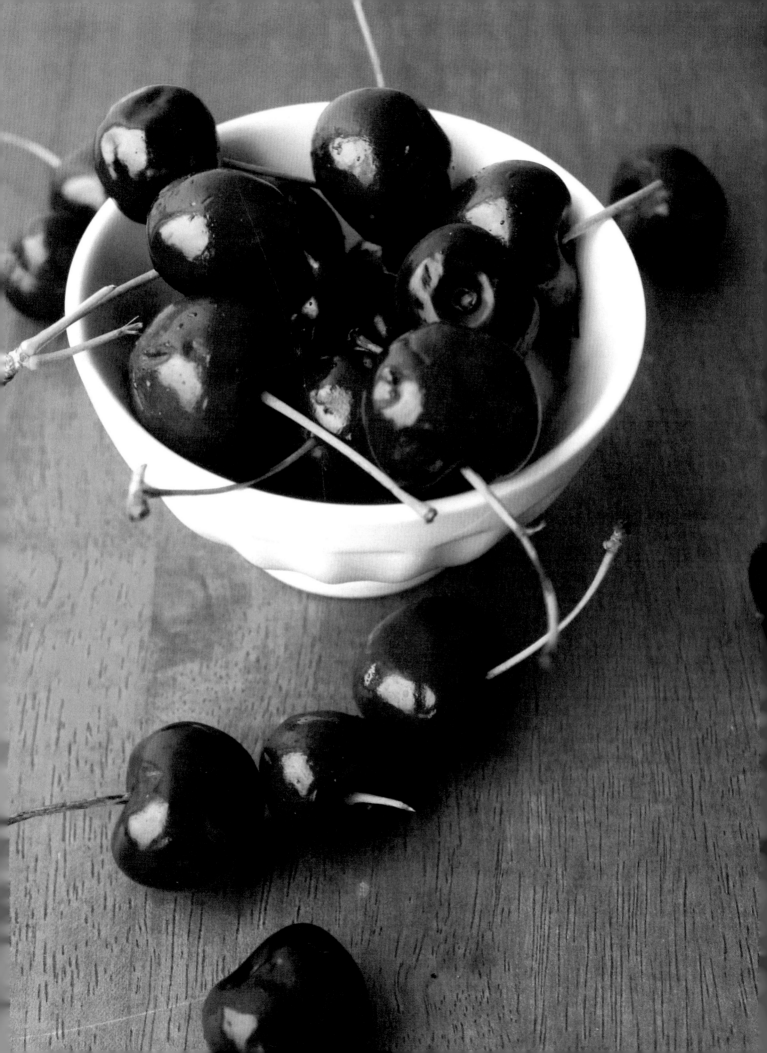

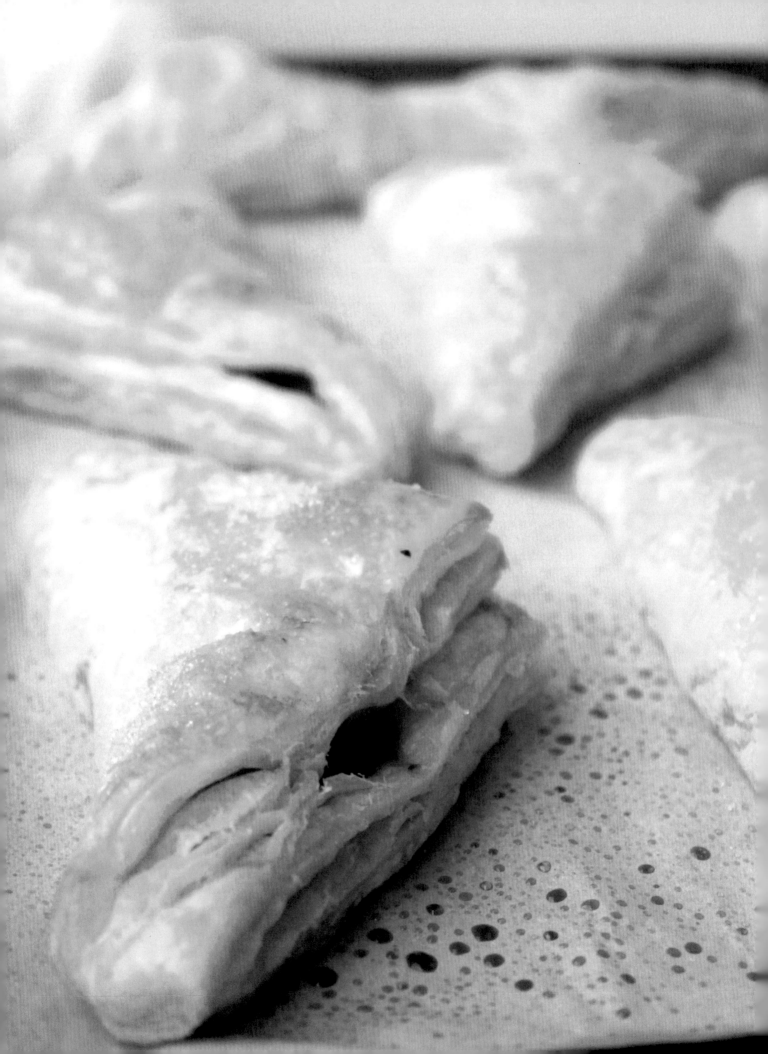

Cherry Turnovers

Makes 8 turnovers

1 package puff pastry (2 sheets)

16 cherries, pitted and cut in quarters

1 tbsp butter or margarine, melted

Sugar, for dusting

Thaw puff pastry sheets according to package directions. Lay each sheet out on a cutting board, then cut into 4 equal squares. Put an equivalent of 2 whole cherries onto each square, then fold in half diagonally, sealing edges shut. Repeat for the rest of the turnovers.

Heat oven to 350 F. Put parchment paper on a large baking sheet, then arrange all the turnovers so they are not touching. Brush butter on top of each, then sprinkle with sugar. Bake 10-12 minutes or until golden on top. Serve warm.

Boozy Cherries over Ice Cream

Serves 4

1/2 lb cherries, pitted

1/4 c. sugar

1 quart mason jar

Your favorite vodka or other liquor

Combine cherries and sugar in the mason jar, then top with your favorite vodka. I love to use chocolate vodka, but any citrus or berry flavor would work as well. Let marinate in the refrigerator for at least a day before serving. Spoon cherries over ice cream to serve.

Bonus: Pour chilled vodka into a martini glass for a cherry flavored drink, using a cherry as a garnish.

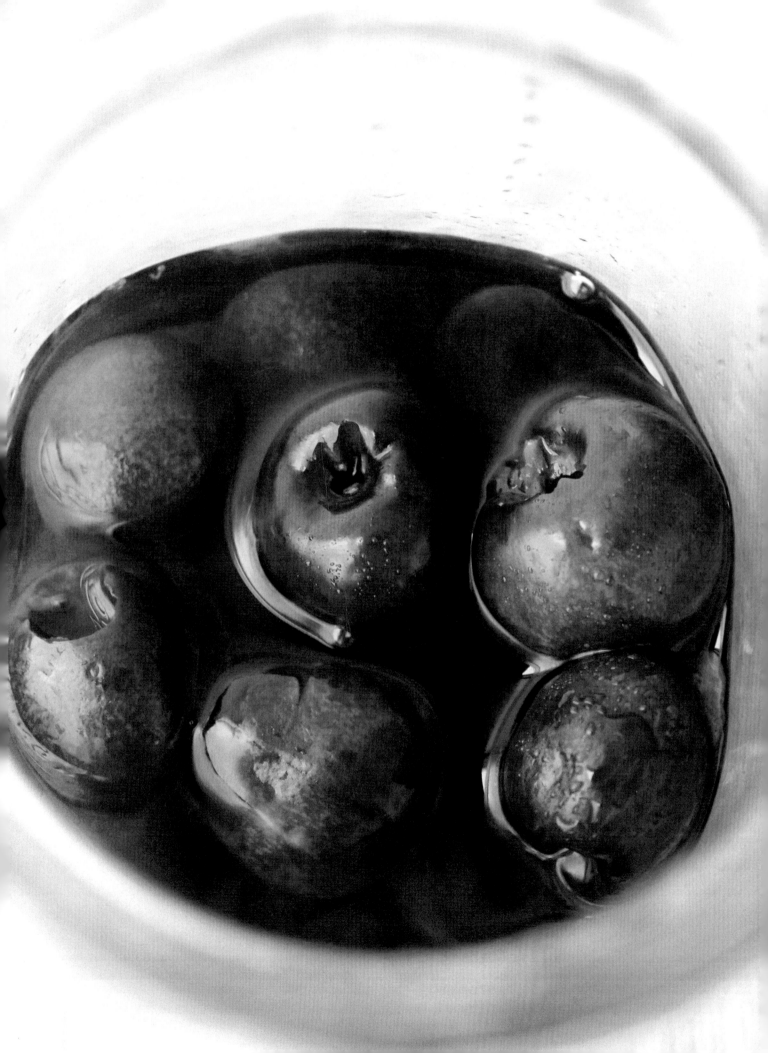

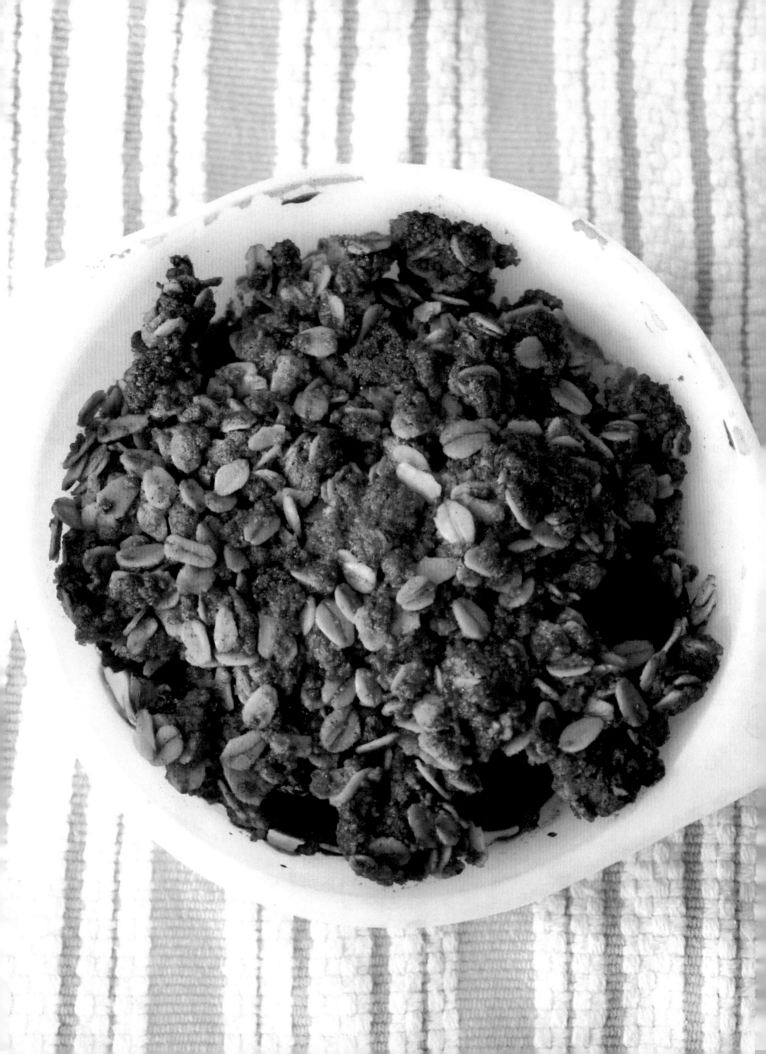

Cinnamon Cherry Crisp

Makes 2 servings

12 cherries

1/2 c. regular rolled oats

2 tbsp flour

2 tbsp brown sugar

1/2 tsp cinnamon

2 tbsp butter or vegan butter, melted

Preheat oven to 400 F. Add cherries to a small ceramic baking dish. In a medium bowl, combine oats, flour, sugar and cinnamon. Pour melted butter over the top and toss to combine. Pour over the cherries making sure every cherry has some of the oat mixture over it. Bake for 20 minutes until hot and bubbly with a nice crispy crust. Serve by itself or with some vanilla ice cream.

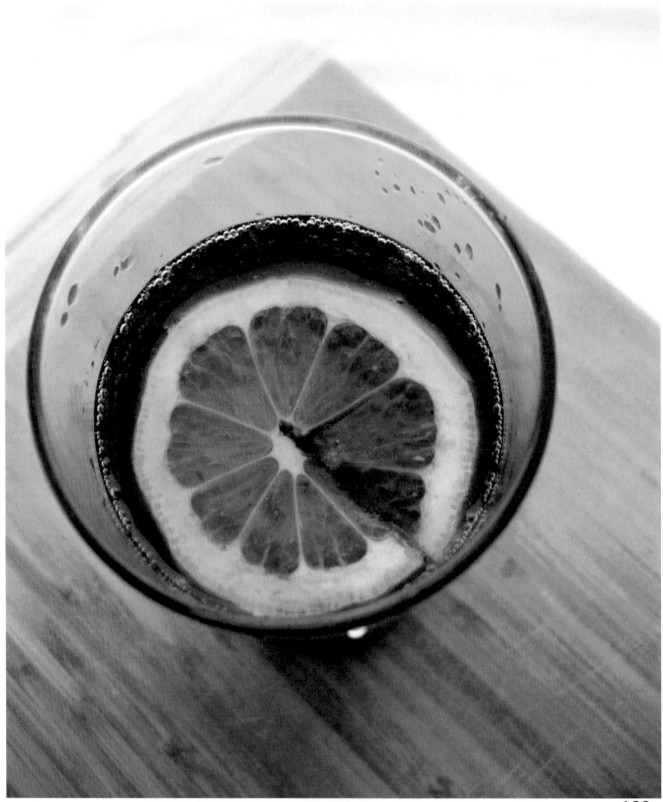

Cherry Lemon Soda

Makes 1 drink

4 oz. cherry juice (preferably Bing)

1 tbsp lemon juice

1 tbsp simple syrup

1 oz. vodka, optional

ice

sparkling water

lemon slice, for garnish

Stir together cherry juice, lemon juice, simple syrup and vodka in a tall glass. Add ice, then fill to top with sparkling water. Garnish with lemon slice.

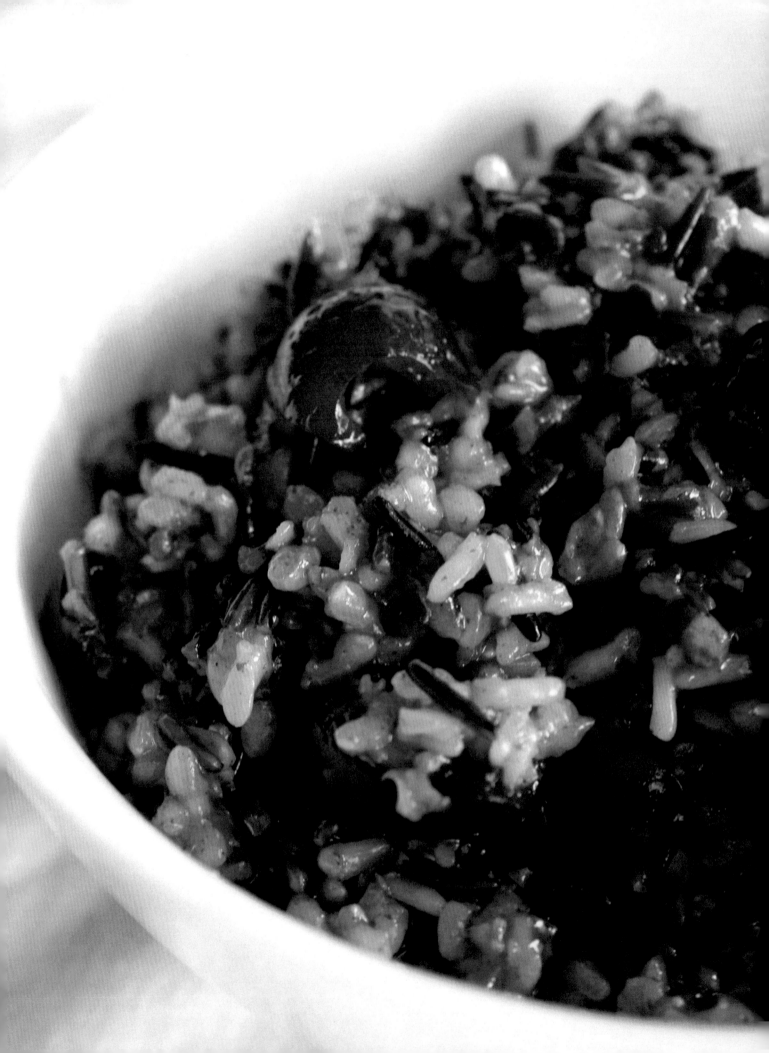

Cherry Studded Wild Rice Pilaf

Serves 4

1 c. wild rice

1 sweet onion, diced

1 clove garlic, minced

2 c. beef or vegetable stock

1 tsp ground sage

1/2 tsp salt

1/4 tsp pepper

12 cherries, pitted and cut in half

In a medium saucepan, heat 1 tbsp olive oil over medium heat. Add onions and garlic and sauté for 2 minutes. Add wild rice and stir to coat in oil. Add stock and spices. Bring to a boil, then reduce to a simmer and cook for 45-50 minutes, or according to package directions.

Once rice is cooked, stir in cherries and serve hot.

Limes

Lemons and limes. Those citrus fruits that are so great in everything, from sorbets and cocktails to cakes and cream pies. Not much says summer more than these two citrus fruits.

Limes are especially delicious when paired with more Mexican flavors, but they really go well with anything, sweet or savory. My favorite lime recipe is the cilantro lime steak. The sauce is so perfectly summery and goes great on any grilled meat. Served with a nice salad and some crunchy bread, it makes a perfect summer meal.

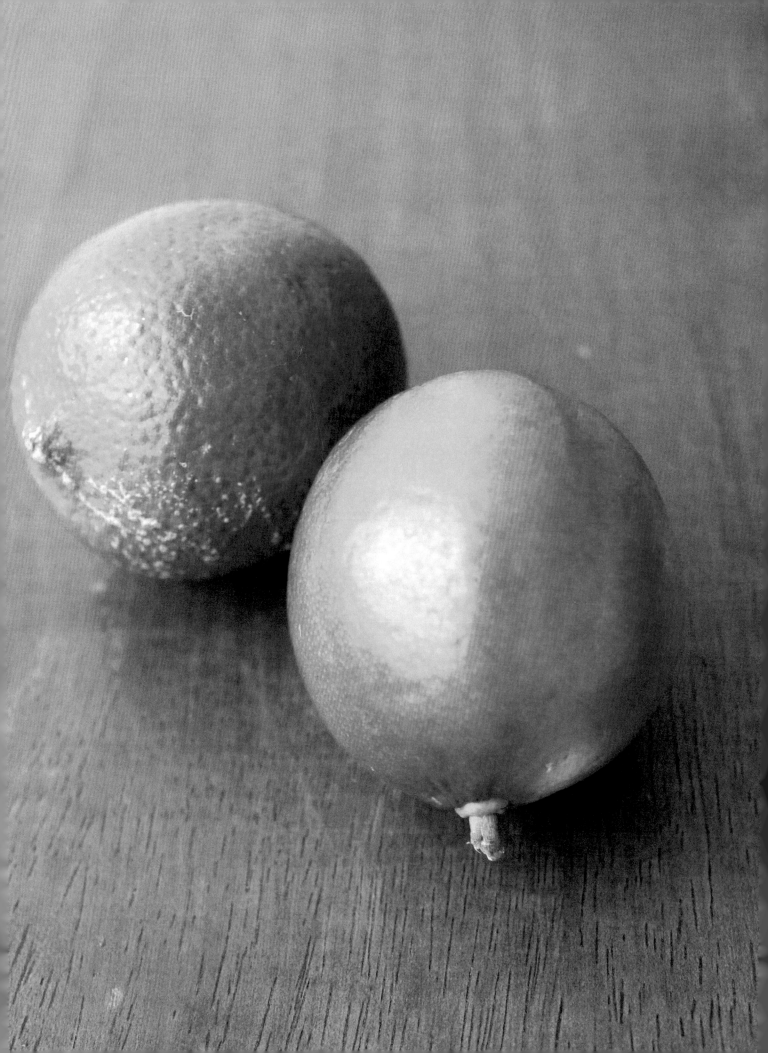

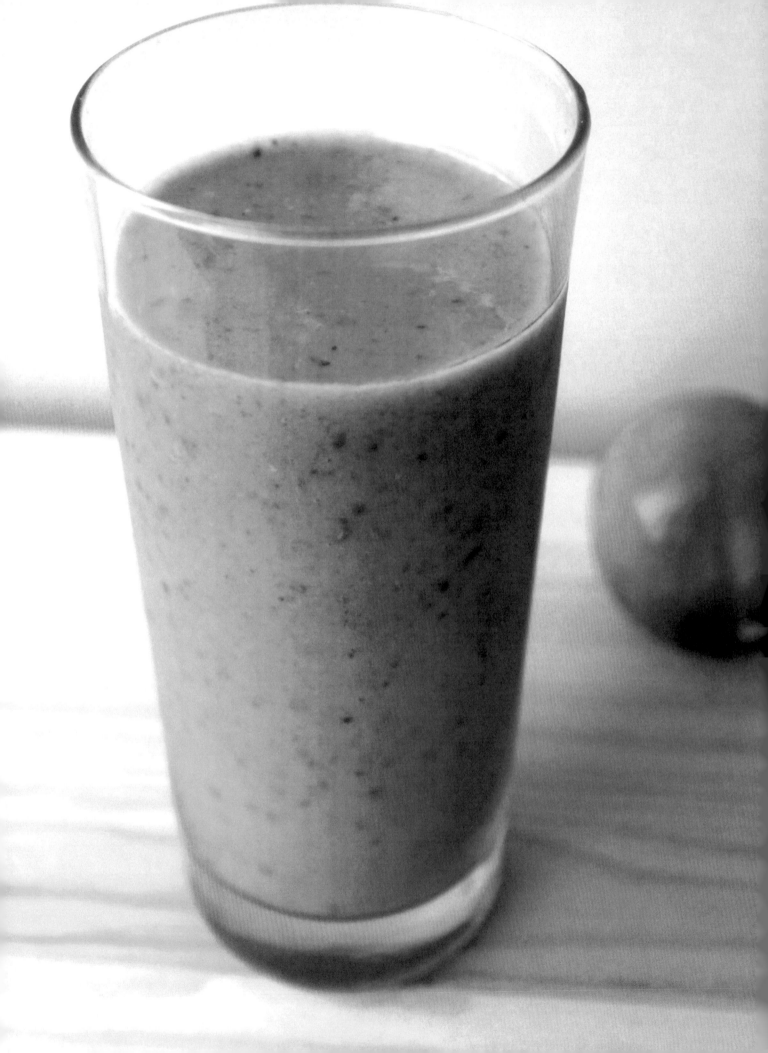

Lime and Raspberry Smoothie

Makes 1 smoothie

1 c. frozen raspberries

Zest of 1 lime

Juice of ½ lime

1 c. almond milk

5 ice cubes

1 tsp agave syrup, if desired

Add all ingredients to a blender and puree until smooth. Serve in a tall glass.

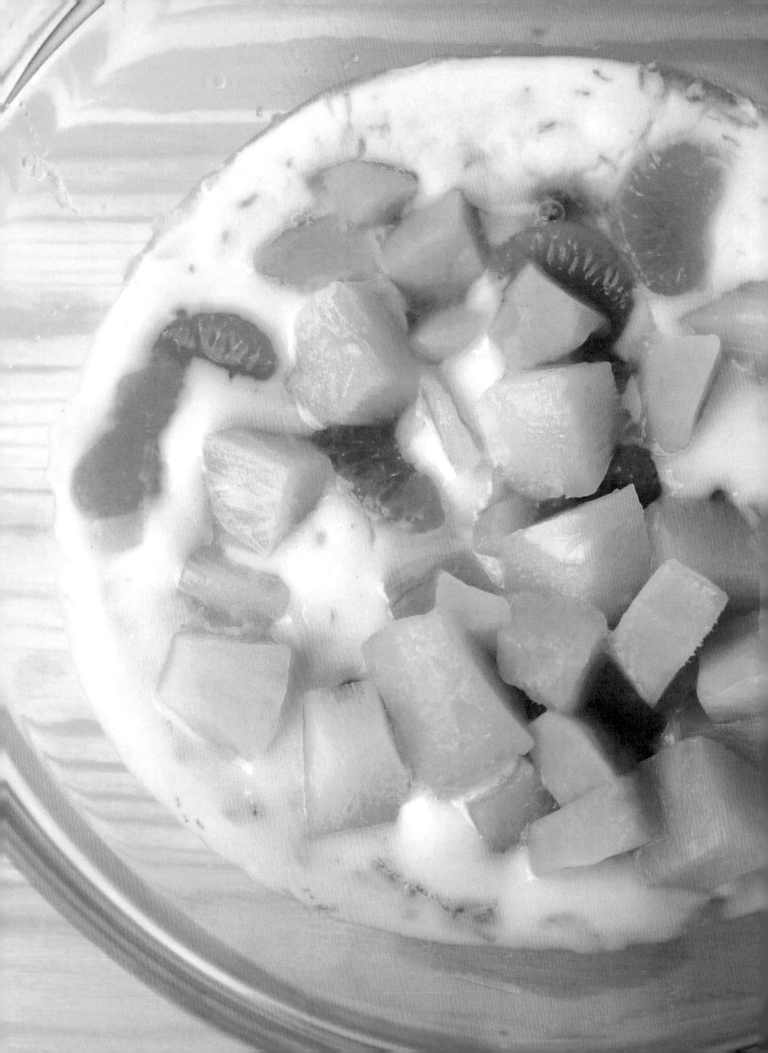

Lime Yogurt with Tropical Fruits

Serves 4

2 containers plain coconut yogurt

Zest of 1 lime

Juice of 1 lime

1 can pineapple chunks, drained

1 small can mango chunks, drained

1 small can mandarin orange slices, drained

In a large bowl, mix together yogurt, lime zest and lime juice. Spoon into 4 bowls, then top each with a mixture of pineapple, mango and orange slices.

Bonus: Mix together pineapple, mango and orange juices from cans and blend in a blender with ice cubes for a tropical slushy.

Lime Mint Shaved Ice with Watermelon

Serves 4

2 c. store bought limeade

1/2 c. sugar

1 handful mint, chopped

Watermelon chunks

Combine limeade and sugar and chopped mint. Pour into a container and set into the freezer to firm up, stirring every couple of hours.

To serve, put some watermelon chunks into a bowl, then shave ice crystals from the lime mint frozen ice cube using a spoon, and sprinkle over the watermelon chunks.

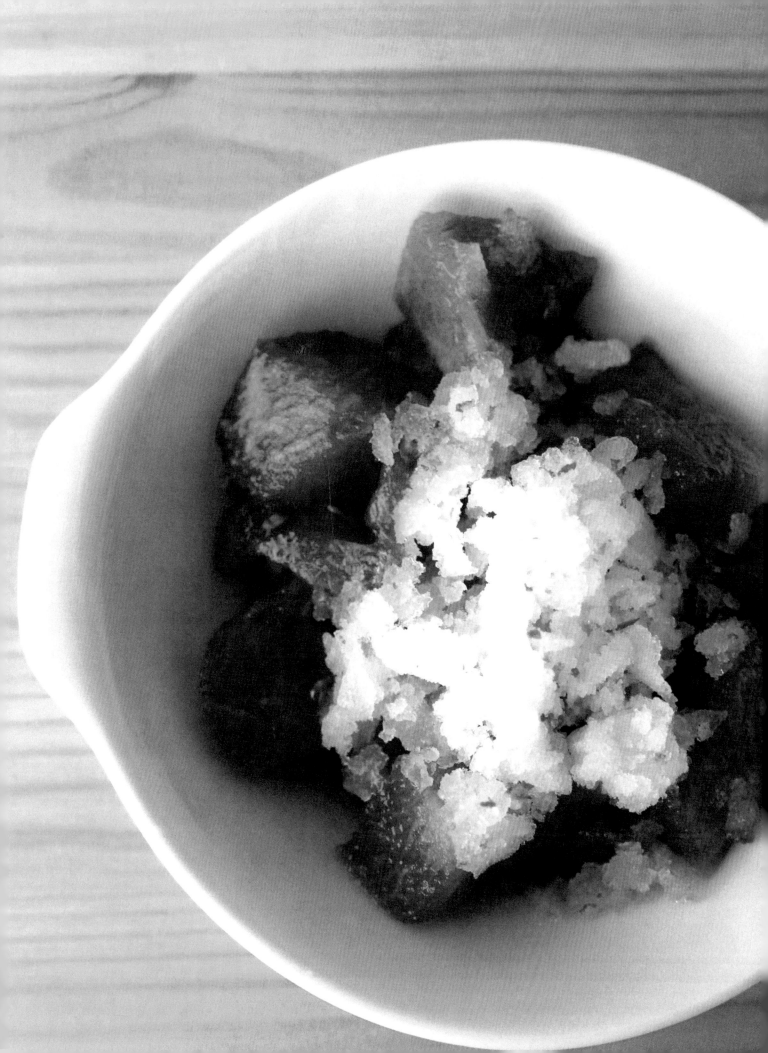

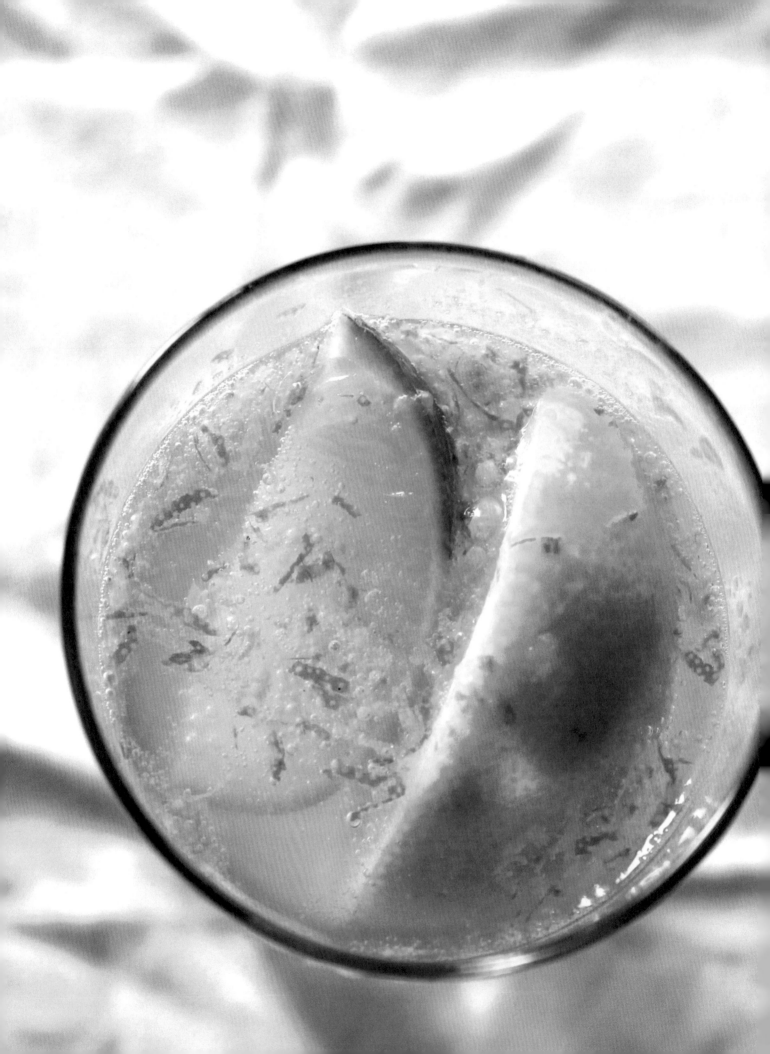

Homemade Lemon Lime Soda

Makes 2 drinks

Zest of 1 lime and 1 lemon

Juice of 1 lime and 1 lemon

4 tbsp simple syrup

Sparkling water

In each glass, put half of the zests and juices, then add 2 tbsp simple syrup in each glass. Stir to mix, then fill with sparkling water.

Cilantro Lime Steak

Serves 4

Your favorite cut of steak

Juice and zest of 1 lime

1/2 bunch green onions, sliced

Handful cilantro

1/4 c. olive oil

1/2 tsp salt

1/4 tsp pepper

Heat a large sauté pan over medium high heat. Sprinkle with salt and pepper, and sear steak, turning once. After steaks are cooked to your liking, set aside and keep warm.

Meanwhile, in a food processor combine lime juice and zest, green onions and cilantro. Process until chopped finely. Add olive oil, salt and pepper and process until emulsified. Pour dressing over steaks and serve with corn and potatoes.

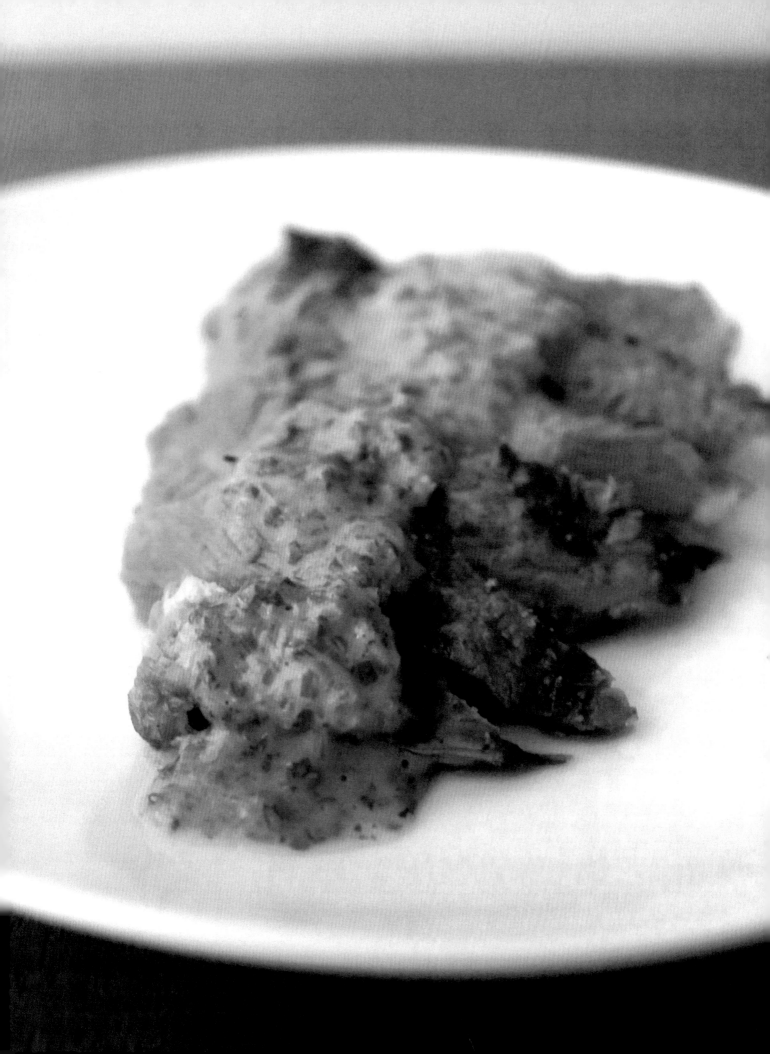

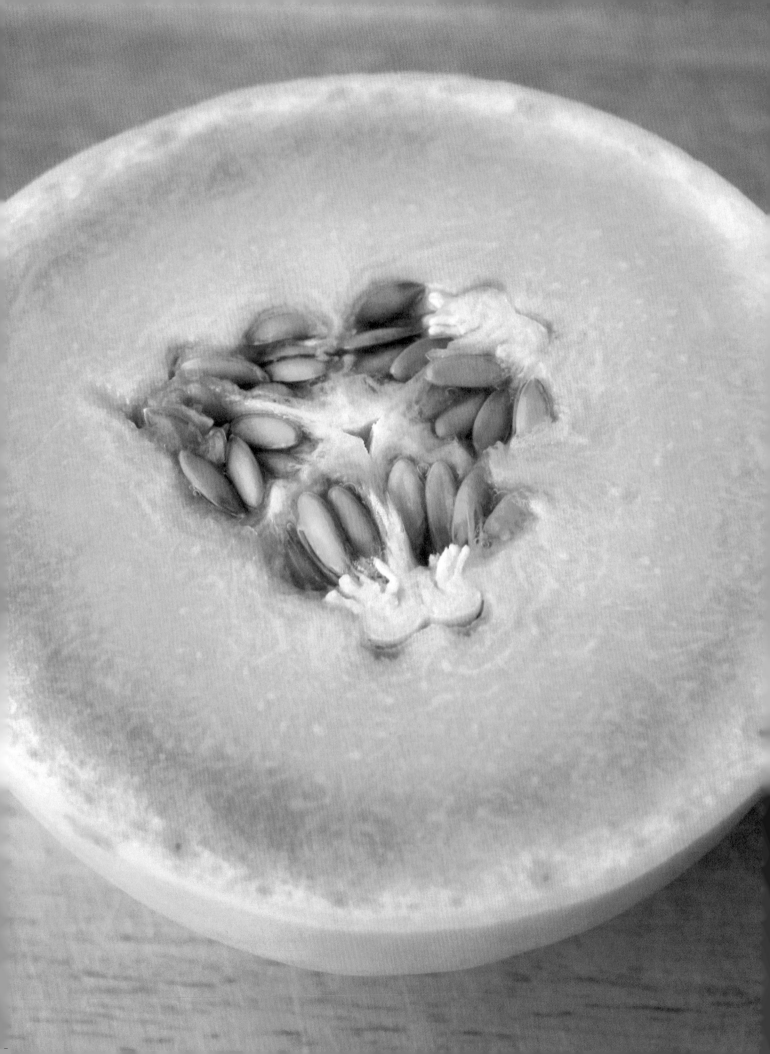

Melons

Most of the time, melons are usually served simple, cut into chunks and typically combined into a nice fruit dish. There is absolutely nothing wrong with enjoying the sweet watery goodness of a melon, especially those that are fresh cut, but I wanted something a little more.

I spiced up some melons in several salads, and made two drinks that are so worthy of your picnic table. The best recipe in this section is the honeydew lemonade. It's made so simply, but the honeydew adds an extra splash of sweetness I just can't resist.

Honeydew Salad with Lime and Mint

Serves 4

1 medium honeydew, cut into chunks or roughly 3 c. chopped honeydew

Juice and zest of 1 lime

1 tsp sugar or agave syrup

Handful of mint leaves, chopped

Mix together lime juice, zest and sugar or syrup in a large bowl. Add mint leaves and honeydew chunks, then toss to combine with dressing. Leave to marinate at room temperature for 30 minutes before serving.

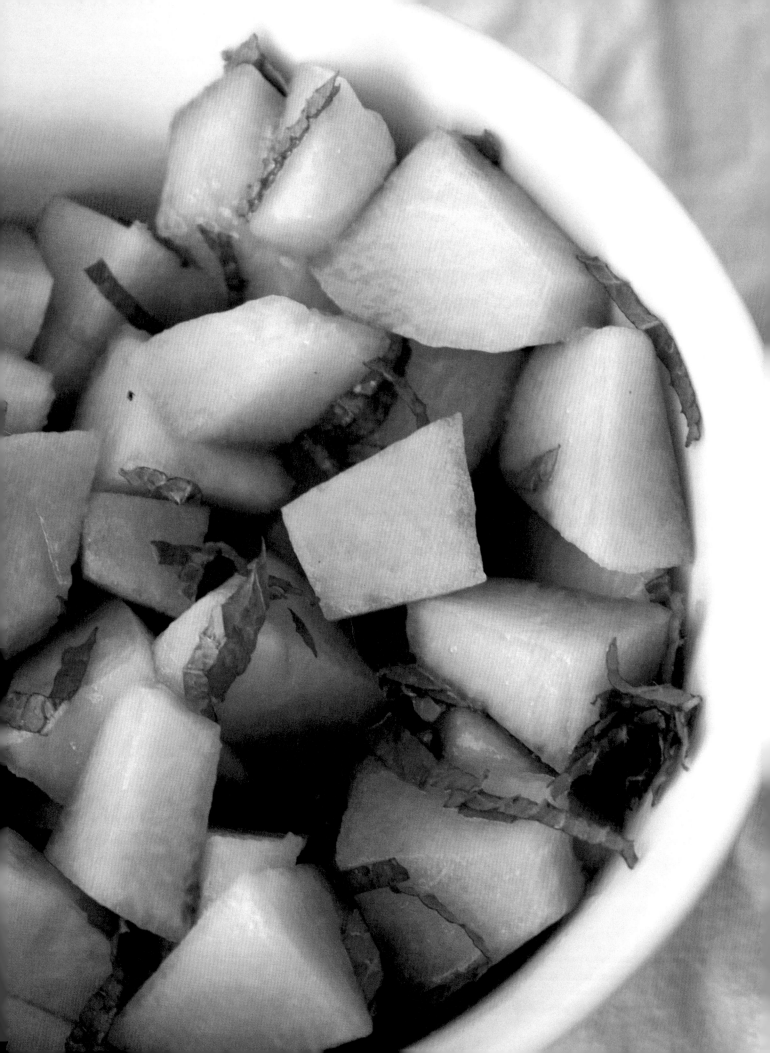

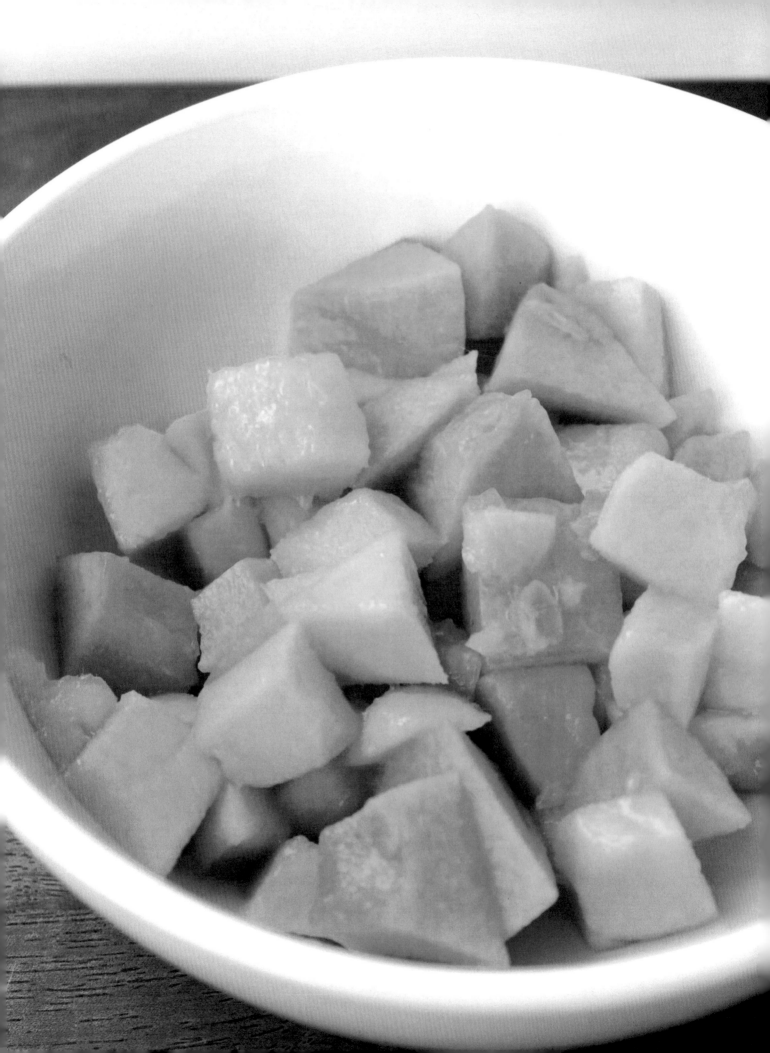

Cantaloupe and Mango Salad

Serves 4

½ medium cantaloupe, rind removed and flesh diced

1 large mango, peeled and diced

Juice of 1 lime

1 tbsp crystallized ginger

In a large bowl, mix lime juice and ginger. Let stand while chopping the fruit. Add the mango and cantaloupe chunks, stir, then cover and chill for at least 3 hours before serving.

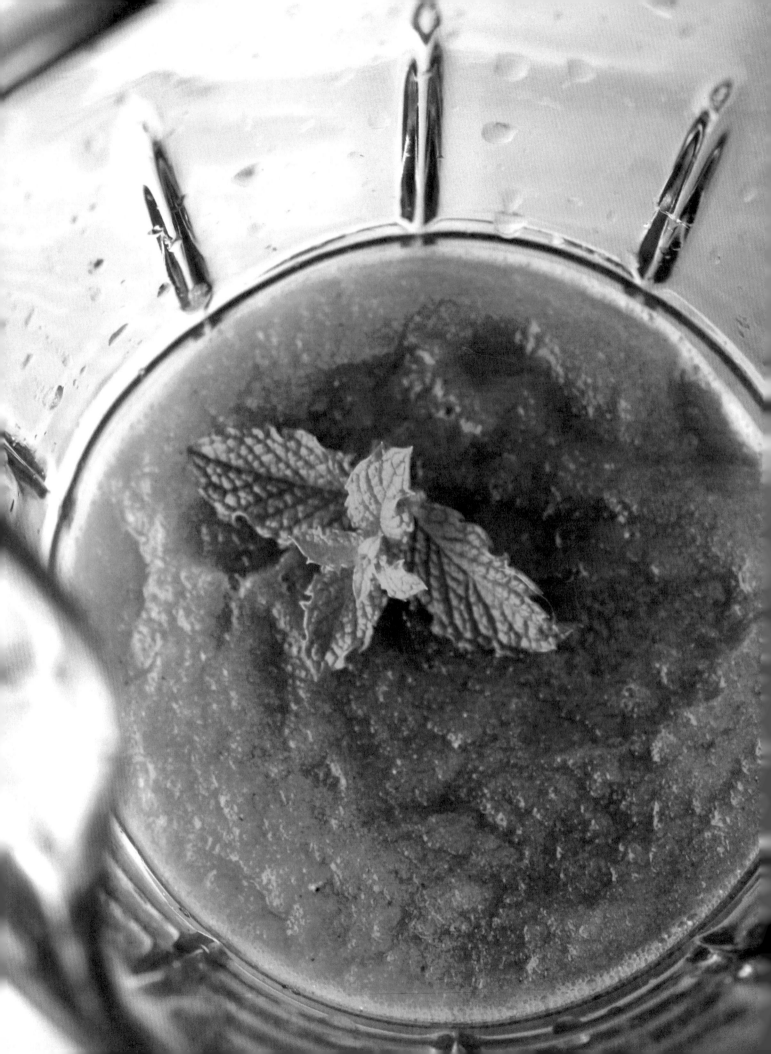

Watermelon Slushy

Makes 4 drinks

5 c. cubed watermelon

2 c. cubed ice

4 oz vodka, if desired

8 mint leaves, plus extra for garnish

4 basil leaves

In a blender, combine all ingredients. Blend until ice cubes are broken up and the consistency is like a slushy. Serve in tall glasses with a few mint leaves for garnish.

Honeydew and Basil Lemonade with Rum

Serves 1

1 c. chopped honeydew

1/2 c. store bought lemonade

1 large basil leaf

1 oz. rum, optional

Ice

In a blender, puree honeydew with lemonade and basil. Strain mixture through a sieve, then pour into a cocktail shaker. Add a few cubes of ice and rum, if using, and shake a few times to blend and chill. Pour into a large glass and serve.

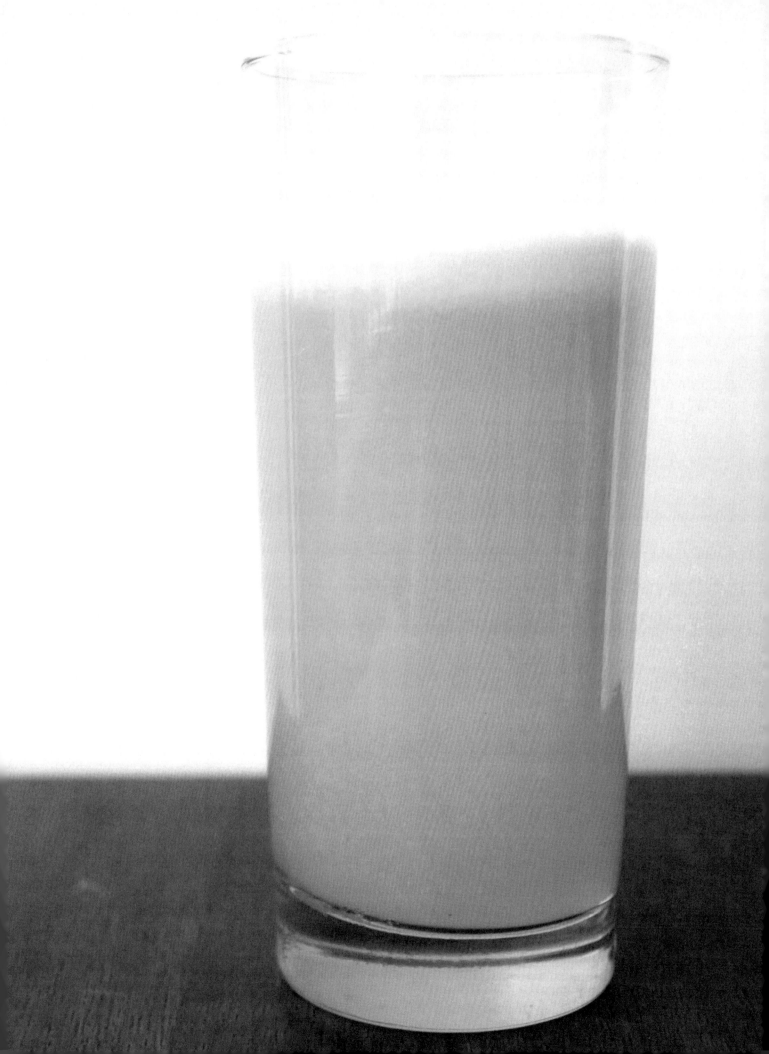

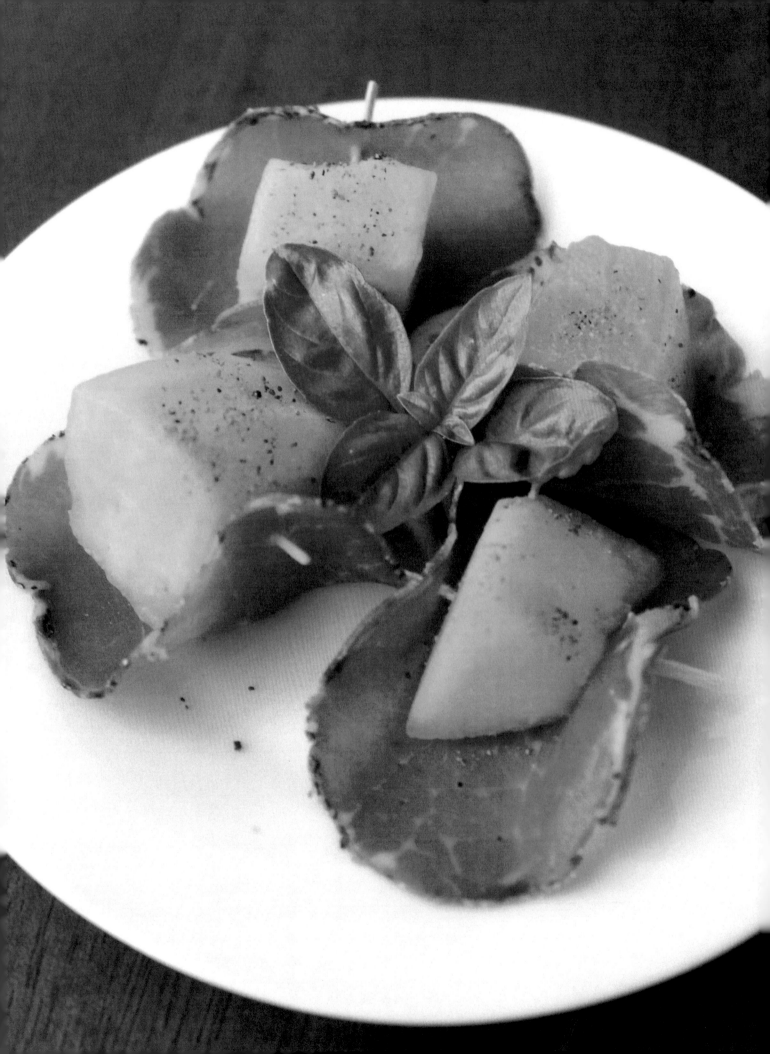

Cantaloupe and Coppa Bites

Makes 12 bites

1 1/2 c. cubed cantaloupe, or roughly 12 cubes

12 slices of coppa or any salami

Nutmeg

12 small basil leaves

toothpicks

On a large plate, lay out the coppa or salami sliced. Put a cube of cantaloupe on each sliced and sprinkle with a dash of nutmeg. Top each with a basil leaf, then spear with a toothpick, wrapping as much of the coppa around the cantaloupe as possible. Serve at room temperature.

Peaches and Nectarines

Peaches are the fuzzier versions of nectarines, but they are both delicious to me. There are no so many varieties available now, from white to yellow to even hybrids, but any will do for me. I especially love it when the nectarines or peaches are so ripe and sweet that you have to eat them over the sink, otherwise the juices will dribble all down your arms and make an absolute delicious mess.

The peach and chicken tacos have always been a hit in my kitchen. I have been making variations of them for years, but this one is my favorite. It's so simple, yet so delicious and can be ready in no time flat. They are perfect for any weeknight dinner rush.

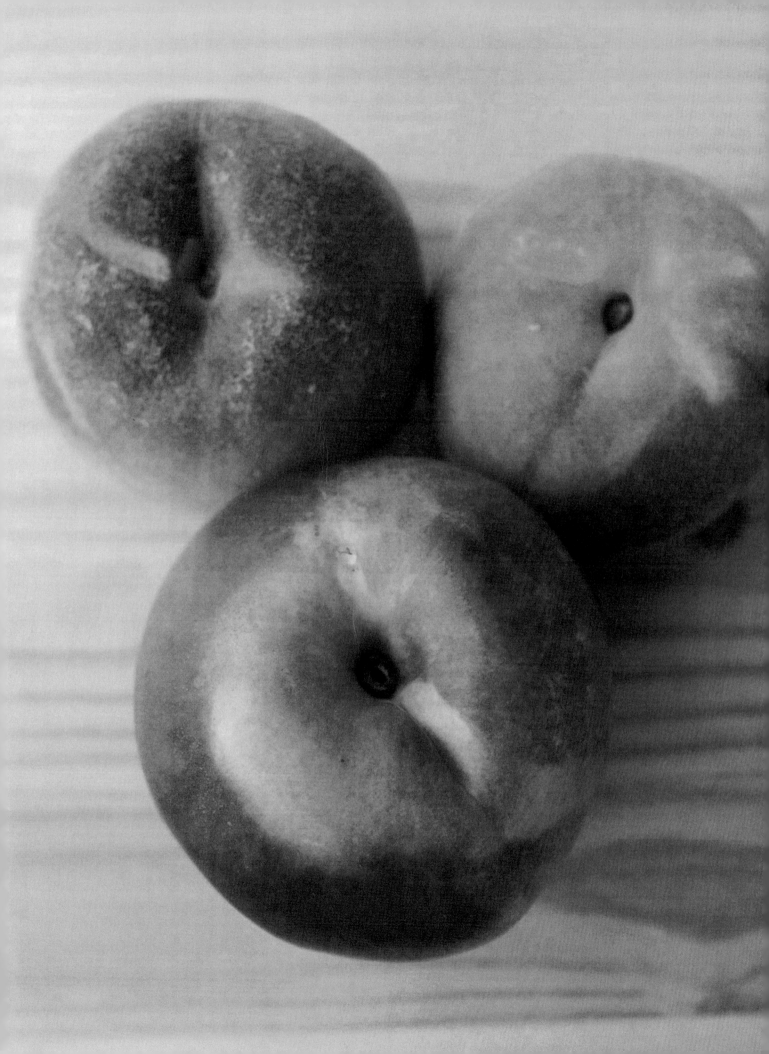

Biscuits with Stewed Ginger Peaches

Makes 12 biscuits

Stewed Peaches:

2 peaches, peeled and diced

1 tsp grated fresh ginger

1/4 tsp allspice

1/4 c. sugar

1/4 c. water

Biscuits:

2 c. AP flour

1 tbsp baking powder

2 tsp sugar

1/2 tsp cream of tartar

1/4 tsp salt

6 tbsp butter or vegan butter (I used Earth Balance)

2 tbsp vegetable shortening

2/3 c. almond milk

In a medium saucepan, combine all ingredients for the peaches. Bring to a boil over medium high heat, then reduce to a simmer and cover. Cook for 20 minutes until peaches being to fall apart. Set aside to cool.

Meanwhile, make the biscuits. Preheat oven to 450 F. Combine flour, baking powder, sugar, cream of tartar and salt in a large bowl. Cut in butter and shortening with a pastry blender or two knives until butter is the size of peas or smaller. Pour all of the milk into the batter and mix together using a fork until just moistened. (There will still be some dry ingredients that don't get mixed in and that's ok).

Pour dough onto a lightly floured surface and knead 4 to 5 times just to combine the dough a little better. Roll the dough out to 1/2" thick then cut dough with a 2.5" cookie cutter. Place biscuits on an ungreased baking sheet with room between them and bake for 10 minutes or until golden brown. Let cool then enjoy with stewed peaches.

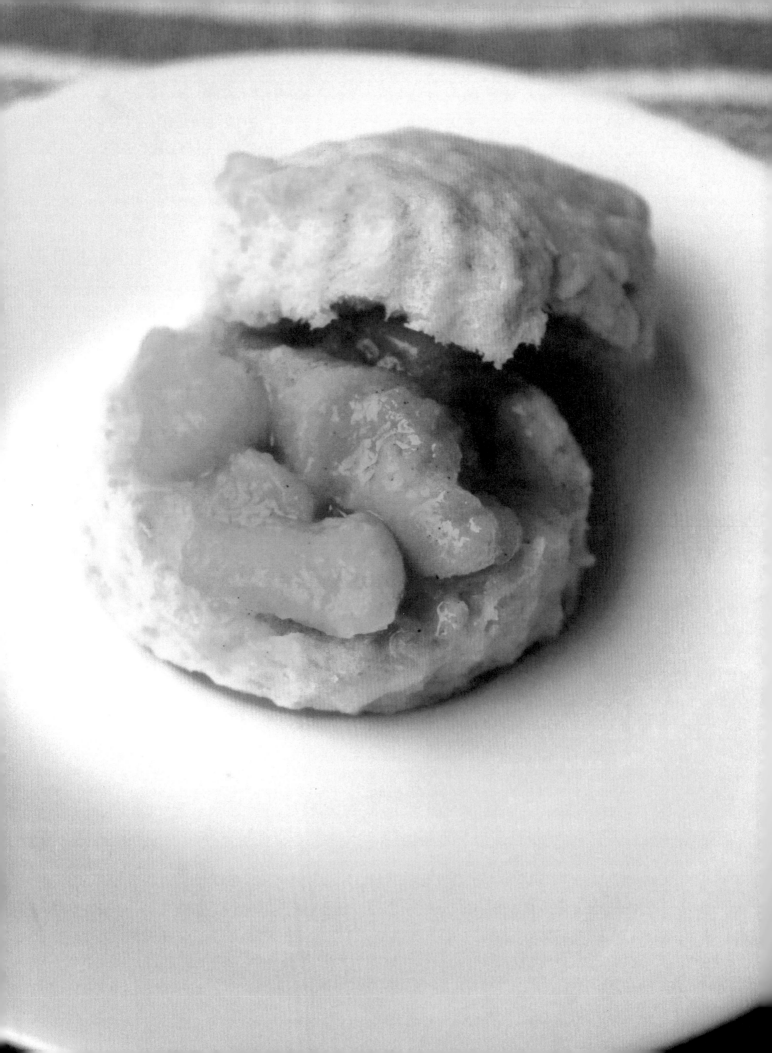

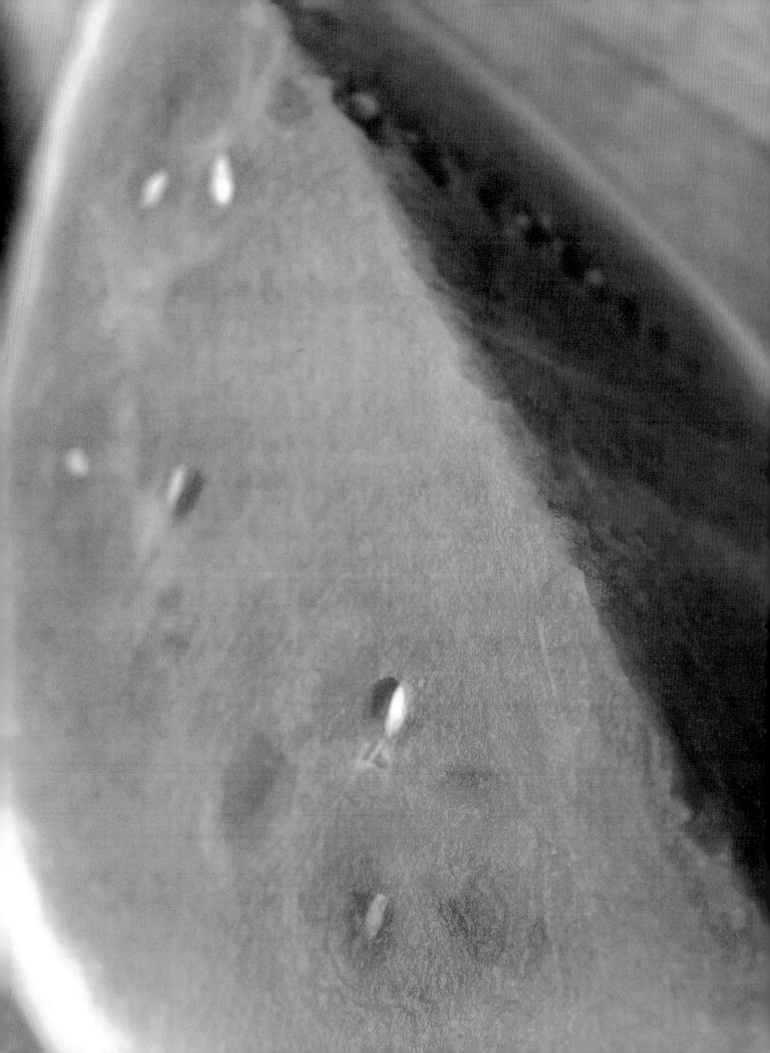

Stone Fruit Salad

Serves 4

1 1/2 lb. stone fruits (I used 1 plum, 2 peaches and 2 apricots)

1/2 c. plus 1/4 c. apricot nectar

1 tbsp cornstarch

1 tbsp honey

10 mint leaves, chopped

To prepare stone fruit, cut each in half, then remove the pit. Cut each half into 3-4 wedges, then put into a large bowl.

In a medium saucepan, bring 1/2 c. apricot nectar to a boil. In a small bowl, whisk together 1/4 c. apricot nectar with cornstarch to make a slurry, then add to boiling apricot nectar. Add honey and let bubble for 1 min. Remove from heat, then pour over fruit.

Sprinkle chopped mint leaves over the top and toss to combine. Cover with plastic wrap and chill for at least an hour before serving.

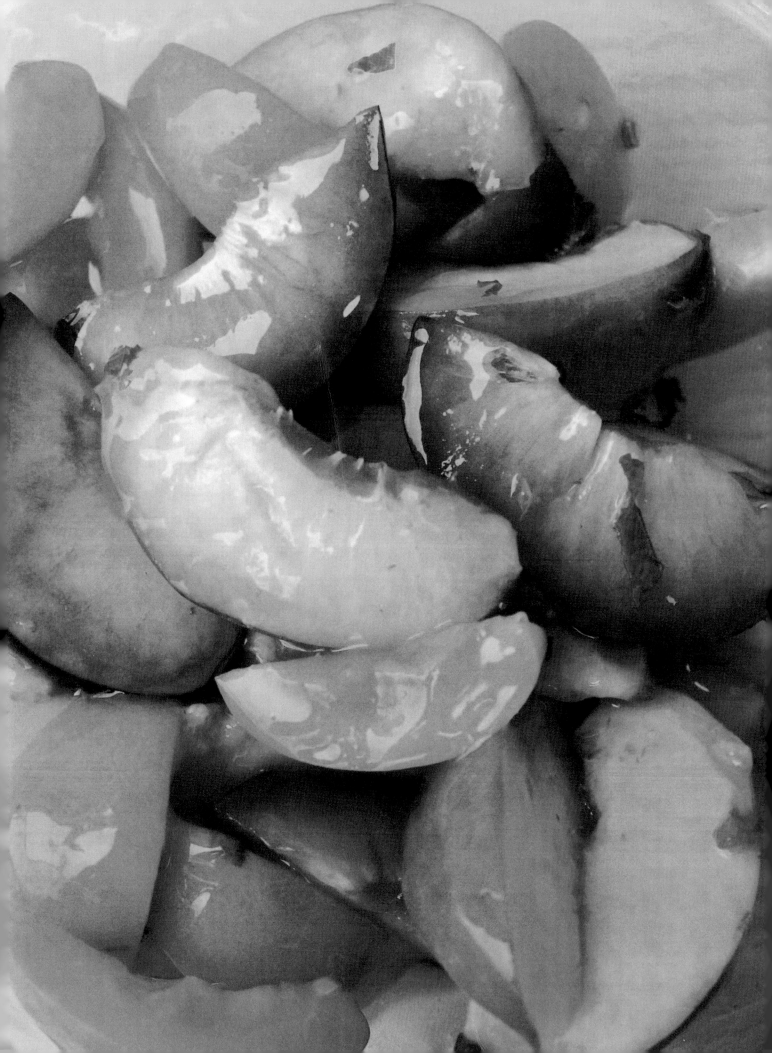

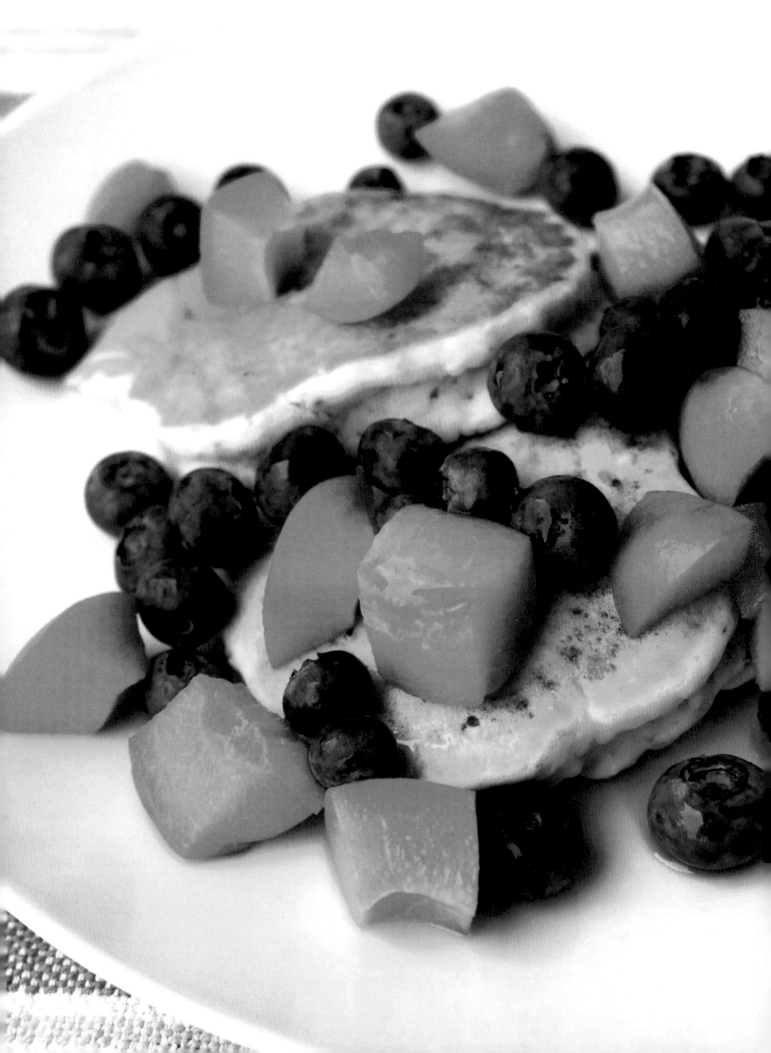

Nectarines and Blueberries over Pancakes

Serves 4

1/2 c. all-purpose flour

1/2 c. whole wheat flour

1 tbsp sugar

1 tsp baking powder

1/4 tsp baking soda

1/4 tsp salt

1 tbsp chia seeds

1 c. almond milk

2 tbsp cooking oil

2 nectarines, pitted and diced

1/2 pint blueberries, rinsed

Maple syrup

In a small bowl, mix together chia seeds with 3 tbsp water. Let stand for 2-3 minutes before using.

In another bowl, mix together flours, sugar, baking powder, baking soda and salt. Add almond milk and cooking oil to the chia seeds, then pour into the flour. Mix well until there are few lumps left.

Heat a skillet over medium heat. Add 1/4 c. of batter to the pan. Cook for 2-3 minutes until bubbles form on top. Flip and cook for 2 minutes on the other side. Remove from pan and repeat until batter has been used up. Top each pancake with some diced nectarines and a few blueberries. Drizzle with maple syrup, if desired.

Nectarine and Apricot Sangria

Serves 4

2 nectarines, cut into wedges

1 c. apricot nectar

2 tbsp sugar

1 bottle dry white wine (I like Pinot Gris)

In a large pitcher or 1 L glass decanter, combine all ingredients. Use the handle of a wooden spoon to stir, then refrigerate for at least 3 hours before serving. Serve chilled in wine glasses.

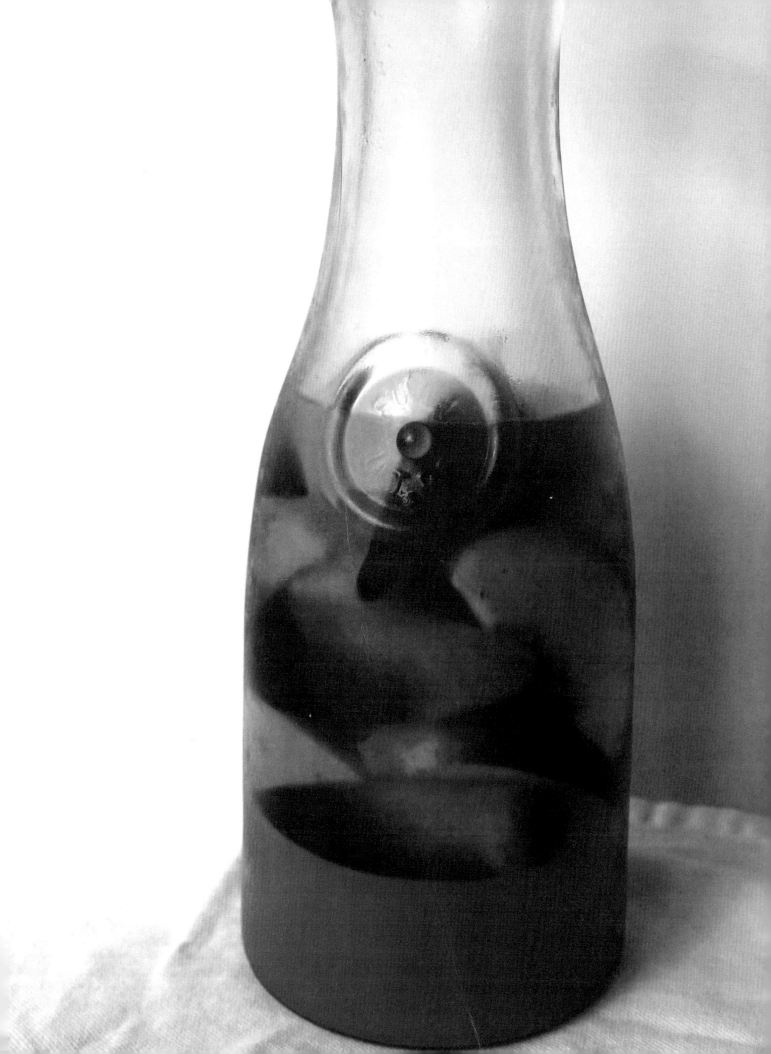

Peach and Chicken Tacos

Serves 4

2 chicken breasts, cut into 1/2" thick strips

1 tsp each chili powder and cumin

1/2 tsp salt

1/4 tsp pepper

2 peaches or nectarines, pitted and cut into slices

1 red bell pepper, cut into strips

1/2 sweet onion, cut in half, then sliced

Tortillas

Combine spices in a bowl, then coat chicken strips. Heat a grill pan or sauté pan over medium high heat. Cook chicken, tossing every minute or so, for a total of 4-5 minutes. Set aside.

Add bell peppers and onions to pan and cook for 3-4 minutes until onions begin to get soft. Add peach slices and sauté for 2 more minutes. Add chicken to reheat, then serve hot with warm tortillas.

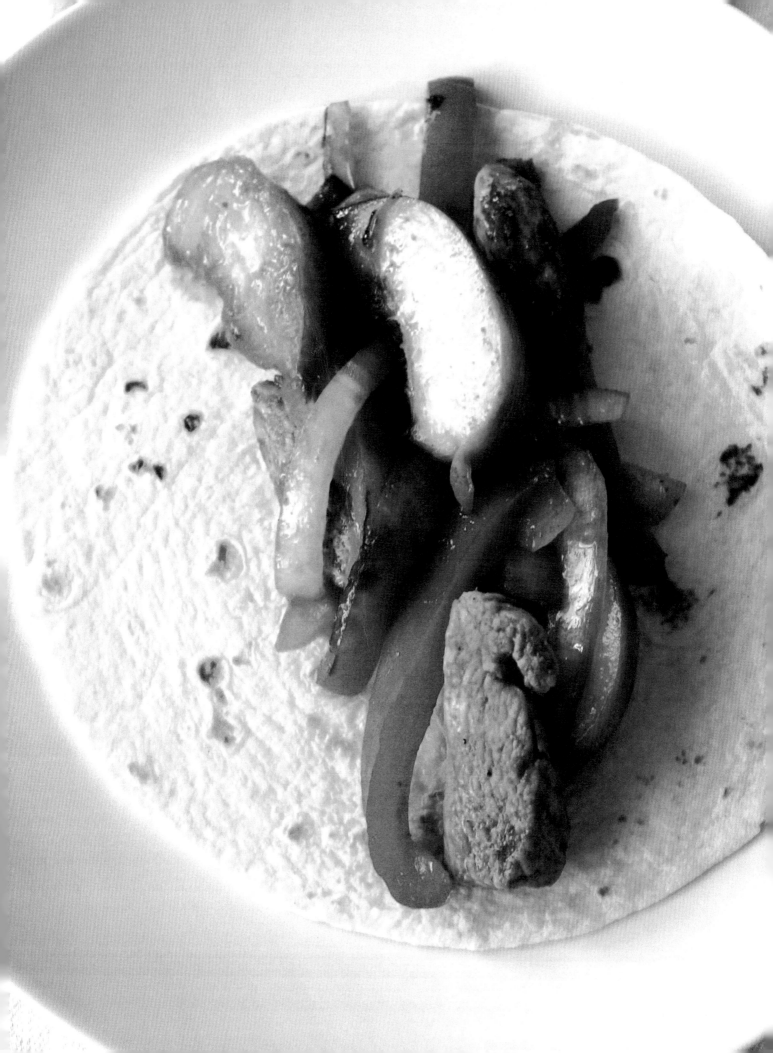

Allergy Notes

All recipes either have no dairy or eggs or are easily modified for those with dairy and egg allergies. Those that have options for dairy and/or eggs include the alternatives in the recipes. Many recipes are gluten free as long as they are made with certified gluten free ingredients.

Index by dish

Appetizers
Asian Crab Salad on
Cucumber Slices   11
Cantaloupe and Coppa
Bites   147
Green Bean Spring Rolls   22
Marinated Dill Mustard
Tomatoes on Crostini   63
Summer Squash and
Parmesan on Crostini   50

Salads
Greek Salad over Romaine   45
Grilled Romaine Caesar Salad
43
Grilled Steak Salad with Corn
47
Roasted Veggie Salad with
Crab   29
Summer Simple Salad   76

Sandwiches
Bacon, Kale, Tomato, Avocado
and Crab   67
Cucumber Sandwich with Sun
Dried Tomato Goat Cheese
Spread   15
Grilled Summer Squash and
Chicken Sandwich with Honey
BBQ Sauce   54

Soups
Creamy Dairy-Free Tomato
Soup   64
Cucumber and Mint Soup   12
Summer Squash and Shrimp
Soup with Orzo   53
Zucchini and Quinoa Soup
with Lemon and Thyme   76

Entrees
Beef Stew with Green Beans
26
Blueberry Sauce over Steak
110
Cilantro Lime Steak   134
Fresh Tomato Basil Pasta   71
Hoisin Chicken Lettuce Wraps
39
Peach and Chicken Tacos   160
Risotto with Garlicky Green
Beans and Shrimp   32
Summer Squash Burgers   58
Zucchini Presto Pasta with
Crispy Coppa   85

Sides
Apricot Blueberry Rice Pilaf
98
Baked Zucchini and Tomatoes
with Panko Crust   82
Cherry Studded Wild Rice
123
Chilled Soba Noodles with
Cucumbers   19

Green Beans in Garlic Black Bean Sauce   31
Grilled Corn, Tomato, Zucchini and Sweet Onion Salad   78
Roasted Italian Cherry Tomatoes   69
Summer Squash and Quinoa Pilaf   57

Desserts
Apricot Sugar Cookies with Lavender   93
Blackberry Lemon Cake   107
Boozy Cherries over Ice Cream   116
Cantaloupe and Mango Salad   141
Cinnamon Cherry Crisp   119
Honeydew Salad with Lime and Mint   138
Lime Mint Shaved Ice with Watermelon   130
Lime Yogurt with Tropical Fruits   129
Stone Fruit Salad   154

Breakfasts
Apricot Bread   94
Blackberry Yogurt Fool with Peaches   104
Blueberry Walnut Oatmeal   103
Biscuits with Stewed Ginger Peaches   150
Cherry Turnovers   115
Chocolate Zucchini Bread   75
Lime and Raspberry Smoothie   127

Nectarines and Blueberries over Pancakes   157
Spiced Apricots over Oatmeal   91

Drinks
Apricot Vanilla Soda   97
Black and Blue Martini   109
Cherry Lemon Soda   121
Homemade Lemon Lime Soda   133
Honeydew and Basil Lemonade with Rum   144
Nectarine and Apricot Sangria   158
Watermelon Slushy   143

Condiments
Sweet Dill Homemade Refrigerator Pickles   16

Index by secondary ingredients

Apricot nectar   91, 94, 158
Avocado   67
Bacon   67
Bean threads   22
Beans   64
Beef   58
Bell pepper   45, 54, 85, 160
Blueberries   98, 157
Carrots   22, 26
Chia seeds   157
Chicken   22, 39, 54, 160
Chickpeas   45
Chocolate   75
Ciabatta   54
Corn   26, 46, 78
Crab   11, 29, 67
Crostini   50, 63
Croutons   40, 43
Cucumber   45
Dill   16
Feta   45
Goat cheese   15
Greens   29
Lavender   93
Lemon   107, 121, 133
Lemonade   144
Lime   138
Mango   128, 141
Oats   91, 103, 119

Onion   54, 58, 78
Orange   128
Orzo   53
Panko   79
Parmesan   50
Pasta   71
Peaches   104
Peanut butter   22
Pepperoncini   45
Pineapple   128
Potatoes   26, 29
Puff pastry   115
Quinoa   57, 76
Raspberries   127
Rice   32, 98, 123
Rice paper   22
Salami   85, 147
Shrimp   32, 53
Soba noodles   19
Steak   26, 46, 110, 134
Sun dried tomatoes   15
Tomatoes   29, 40, 45, 46, 78, 79
Water chestnuts   39
Watermelon   130
White wine   158
Yogurt   128

About the author

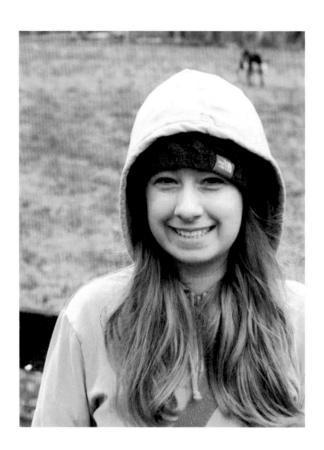

Hello! I'm so glad you picked up my second cookbook. It's been so much of a learning process to write these books, but I have enjoyed every minute of it. A little bit about me then eh? I have been cooking since I could walk, helping my grandma bake cookies or make dumplings. I even did some experimenting without a recipe and ended up with salty hockey pucks, as my grandpa will attest to being force fed several. In addition to doing chemistry in the kitchen, I have had food allergies almost my whole life, and have been dairy and egg free since 2011, which has made my culinary adventure even more exciting.

Outside of the kitchen, I have been skiing since before I was 2, and I still love it. A new love of mine that has cropped up in the past few years is hiking. Growing up in the Puget Sound area has definitely influenced my cooking style, and I plan to stay put. I am working on many more cookbooks, so keep your eyes open for much more.

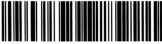

Made in the USA
San Bernardino, CA
21 February 2017